What Should I Eat?

What Should I Eat?

A Complete Guide
to the
New Food Pyramid

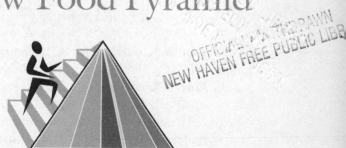

Tershia d'Elgin

BALLANTINE BOOKS NEW YORK

No book can replace the diagnostic expertise and medical advice of a trusted physician. Please be certain to consult with your doctor before making any decisions that affect your health, particularly if you suffer from any medical condition or have any symptom that may require treatment.

2005 Ballantine Books Trade Paperback Edition

Published in the United States by Ballantine Books, an imprint of The Random House Publishing Group, a division of Random House, Inc., New York.

BALLANTINE and colophon are registered trademarks of Random House, Inc.

ISBN 0-345-48743-5

Printed in the United States of America

www.ballantinebooks.com

9 8 7 6 5 4 3 2 1

To Diego Lynch, Louis Hock, and Sam Hock.
Chew On.

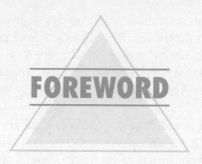

FOREWORD

Today's world is overflowing with nutrition information. How do you determine who and what to believe and how to apply it to you and your situation? As licensed nutritionists and registered dietitians, we know that Americans today often don't know what to eat, drink, or think about their diet, and they don't have time to figure it all out. Most everyone wants to eat better, and to do so, Americans need access to the latest and best nutritional advice. And they need it in a personalized, easy-to-use format.

We are happy to report that *What Should I Eat?* makes the information from the new dietary guidelines easy to understand and workable for everyday life. This book picks up where the website leaves off by making My Pyramid recommendations more usable for everyone, everywhere, all the time—in the grocery store, in the kitchen, and when eating out.

If you do not have a clue about food pyramids or understand why this nutritional counsel is necessary, Chapters 1 and 2 give important background that is not immediately evident at MyPyramid.gov. They tell us how large portions and foods with low nutritional value have affected our population and what good food can do for us. *What Should I Eat?* calls for discerning shopping in the mass market. Chapter 3 gives development background on My Pyramid so you will know how the U.S. Department of Agriculture experts came up with all the new information.

Chapter 4 is the biggie. It tells you all about each of My Pyramid's six food groups—what they are, why they are important, and how much of each you should eat. It makes the benefits of each group easy to grasp and gives some extra nutritional background not found on the website. This chapter also has tips for incorporating more healthful foods into your diet and cutting back on the foods that offer no benefit.

Once you see how these six food groups come together to provide the nutrients to keep you going, then you can move on to thinking about chocolate, ice cream, and french fries. Chapter 5 gives you the lowdown on discretionary calories, describing how many (or how few) extra calories you can afford. If you crave more calories, get ready to burn more, which is the message of Chapter 6.

Chapter 7 is a user's manual for the Nutrient Facts food labels. All those percentages on food packaging can be pretty confusing. Part of getting the maximum nutrient value out of our food depends on careful shopping, storage, and preparation. Chapter 8 contains tips of this sort. Chapter 9 shows how to get big nutrient bang for your restaurant buck. After all, anywhere from one-quarter to one-half of all Americans eat out at least once a day.

Chapter 10 sends you off with a little information about tweaking your proportions to optimize your health, as well as extra suggestions not offered at My Pyramid: adding some vitamin and mineral supplements and getting advice from a registered dietitian to make sure you are on track.

The Resource List is another boost, suggesting good books and websites for learning more about how food makes us run and where to get the freshest foods in your area.

Read on, and when you're through, don't forget to get some exercise!

Susan Mitchell, Ph.D., R.D., L.D./N., F.A.D.A., and
Catherine Christie, Ph.D., R.D., L.D./N., F.A.D.A.
co-authors of *Fat Is Not Your Fate,*
Eat to Stay Young, and *I'd Kill for a Cookie*

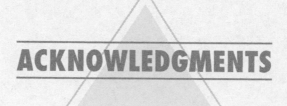

ACKNOWLEDGMENTS

I credit two of the most discriminating women I know with this book: my agent, Julie Castiglia, and my editor, Caroline Sutton. They serve up the kind of guidance that one can never get enough of and friendships that are entirely sating.

Nina Macconnel, Lenore Hughes, Irene de Watteville, and Linas and Susan Naujokaitis—with their ability to mount celebrations for mouths—have taught me the biggest nutrition lesson of my life: that *inferior food and food in the wrong hands is not food.*

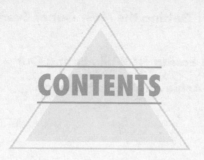

CONTENTS

What Should I Eat?

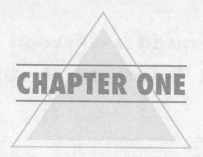

CHAPTER ONE

Why Is a New Food Pyramid Necessary?

A Brief History of Dietary Recommendations

First there was the "square meal," a four-cornered approach to meals that dated from 1943, when the U.S. Department of Agriculture announced the Basic Four to help citizens achieve better nutrition during war shortages. The square meal included a meat portion, a vegetable or fruit portion, a starch portion, and a milk portion, three times a day every day. Baby boomers grew up on square meals. They also grew *out*. By the seventies, Americans were no longer the active, rosy-cheeked specimens depicted in Norman Rockwell illustrations. And as Americans became fatter, scientists proved links between rich food and heart disease. It was obvious that the square meal needed an overhaul.

My Pyramid Is a Product of the USDA, but What Is the USDA?

President Abraham Lincoln created the U.S. Department of Agriculture in 1862. He called it the "people's department." In those days, more than half of all Americans were farmers. Today's statistics are much lower—about 1 percent—yet the USDA still assumes advocacy for the people and corporations that grow our food. At the same time, the USDA is home to the Food, Nutrition, and Consumer Services, whose agencies administer the Center for Nutrition Policy and Promotion. This group links scientific research to consumers' nutritional needs, then distributes science-based dietary guidance. The new My Pyramid is a recent manifestation.

In the late 1970s, the USDA added another category to the Basic Four and put the culprits—sweets, alcohol, and fat—into it. Despite, or perhaps because of, the fifth element, incidences of heart disease, diabetes, hypertension and stroke, and weight gain mounted. So during the eighties the USDA decided to get graphic. The agency came up with an emblem designed to signify what previous polygons could not—*variety, proportion,* and *moderation.* The 1992 Food Pyramid stacked the food groups according to the proportions in which they should be consumed, with grains occupying the wider base and sweets at the top. The message was (and still is), make cereals, rice, pasta, and bread the foundation of your diet. Consume plenty of vegetables and fruits. Enjoy milk, cheese, yogurt, and other dairy

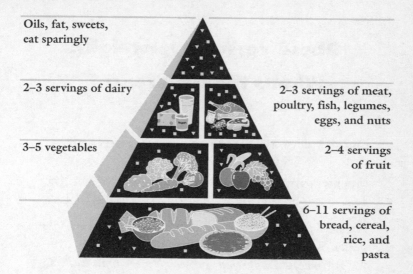

Oils, fat, sweets,
eat sparingly

2–3 servings of dairy

2–3 servings of meat,
poultry, fish, legumes,
eggs, and nuts

3–5 vegetables

2–4 servings
of fruit

6–11 servings of
bread, cereal,
rice, and
pasta

products. Eat some meat, fish, poultry, and legumes. Add a smattering of sweets, oils, and fats.

The old pyramid was more complicated than the square meal, but was still fairly simple. Its advice was also better for us and reflected the growing body of knowledge about carbohydrates, fats, and other components of good nutrition. Unfortunately, it did not make U.S. citizens healthier. Just the opposite.

The Girth Factor

Increasingly poor nutritional habits and lack of exercise undermined the Food Pyramid's good intentions. The pattern of weight gain continued. Of twenty-two industrialized countries, the United States has the highest obesity statistics. Today, fully two-thirds of Americans over the age of twenty are overweight, and nearly one-third of adults are obese, according to the 1999–2000 National Health and Nutrition Examination Survey. This prevalence has increased steadily in the last forty years, in both genders and all ethnic groups. Over these decades, the

Obese versus Overweight: What's the Difference?

OBESITY = ABNORMALLY HIGH PROPORTIONS OF
              BODY FAT

OVERWEIGHT = EXCESS MUSCLE, BONE, FAT, AND/OR
                 BODY WATER RELATIVE TO HEIGHT

All obese people are overweight, but not every overweight person is obese; there is a distinction. Technically, overweight means simply that you weigh more than average. Some people are not fat, but they carry surplus weight in their musculature.

statistics on overweight people increased only marginally (from 32.5 to 33.6 percent), but obesity more than doubled (from 13.3 to 30.9 percent).

If you want to know whether you are overweight and/or obese, use the same system as health professionals and scientists. The *Body Mass Index,* or BMI, can help you determine unhealthy degrees of weight.

Body Mass Index Table

Look at the table on page 8. Find the appropriate height in the left-hand column labeled "Height." Move across to a given weight. The number at the top of the column is the BMI at that height and weight. Pounds have been rounded off.

There are subtleties that indicate just how healthy your BMI is. For instance, bodybuilders and other muscular types

The Body Mass Index Formula

The following equation is based on the metric system:

$$\frac{\text{WEIGHT (KILOGRAMS)}}{\text{HEIGHT (METERS)} \times 2}$$

Using U.S. customary measurements instead, multiply your weight in pounds by 704.5, then divide the result by height in inches, then divide that result by height in inches a second time. Or just use the table.

may be technically overweight but still very fit. However, older people or people who have lost body mass through dieting may fall within a healthy BMI category but have decreased nutritional reserves. There are also distinctions between men and women that are not incorporated into the BMI. Evidently the BMI is not a flawless methodology, but it is the best we have now and it is a good starting place for analysis.

Obesity increases the risk of mortality by 50 to 100 percent. Boiled down, this means that obese people are shortening their lives by anywhere from a handful of years up to twenty years, depending on their BMI.

What about children? Officially, pudgy children are only overweight, not obese. Even though today's children cannot be labeled obese until after they reach the age of twenty, they are, overall, three times as fat as they were thirty-five years ago. In 1970, 4 percent of American children ages 6 through 11 were overweight, as were 5 percent of children ages 12 through 19. Today, 16 percent of all American children carry more weight than they need and more than is healthy. The extra pounds increase their vulnerability to disease and the likelihood that they

BMI Table

						Overweight						Obese									Weight (Pounds)
BMI 19	20	21	22	23	24	25	26	27	28	29	30	31	32	33	34	35	36	37	38	39	40
Height (Inches)																					
58 91	96	100	105	110	115	119	124	129	134	138	143	148	153	158	162	167	172	177	181	186	191
59 94	99	104	109	114	119	124	128	133	138	143	148	153	158	163	168	173	178	183	188	193	198
60 97	102	107	112	118	123	128	133	138	143	148	153	158	163	168	174	179	184	189	194	199	204
61 100	106	111	116	122	127	132	137	143	148	153	158	164	169	174	180	185	190	195	201	206	211
62 104	109	115	120	126	131	136	142	147	153	158	163	169	175	180	186	191	196	202	207	213	218
63 107	113	118	124	130	135	141	146	152	158	163	169	175	180	186	191	197	203	208	214	220	225
64 110	116	122	128	134	140	145	151	157	163	169	174	180	186	192	197	204	209	215	221	227	232
65 114	120	126	132	138	144	150	156	162	168	174	180	186	192	198	204	210	216	222	228	234	240
66 118	124	130	136	142	148	155	161	167	173	179	186	192	198	204	210	216	223	229	235	241	247
67 121	127	134	140	146	153	159	166	172	178	185	191	198	204	211	217	223	230	236	242	249	255
68 125	131	138	144	151	158	164	171	177	184	190	197	203	210	216	223	230	236	243	249	256	262
69 128	135	142	149	155	162	169	176	182	189	196	203	209	216	223	230	236	243	250	257	263	270
70 132	139	146	153	160	167	174	181	188	195	202	209	216	222	229	236	243	250	257	264	271	278
71 136	143	150	157	165	172	179	186	193	200	208	215	222	229	236	243	250	257	265	272	279	286
72 140	147	154	162	169	177	184	191	199	206	213	221	228	235	242	250	258	265	272	279	287	294
73 144	151	159	166	174	182	189	197	204	212	219	227	235	242	250	257	265	272	280	288	295	302
74 148	155	163	171	179	186	194	202	210	218	225	233	241	249	256	264	272	280	287	295	303	311
75 152	160	168	176	184	192	200	208	216	224	232	240	248	256	264	272	279	287	295	303	311	319
76 156	164	172	180	189	197	205	213	221	230	238	246	254	263	271	279	287	295	304	312	320	328

will develop life-threatening illnesses in adulthood, if not before. Just as worrisome are the additional 15 percent who are within a few pounds of joining this category.

The Disease Factor

Americans' problem goes beyond tipping the scale. Many people compromise their health with poor eating habits, even if they are not overweight. Most Americans eat plenty; they just

---

Health Conditions Associated with Poor Eating Habits

DIABETES	COLORECTAL CANCER
HEART DISEASE	KIDNEY CANCER
STROKE	DYSLIPIDEMIA
HYPERTENSION	CONSTIPATION
GALLBLADDER DISEASE	HIGH BLOOD CHOLESTEROL
OSTEOARTHRITIS	
OSTEOPOROSIS	MENSTRUAL IRREGULARITIES
IRON DEFICIENCY ANEMIA	EXCESS BODY AND FACIAL HAIR
SLEEP APNEA AND OTHER BREATHING PROBLEMS	INCONTINENCE
	DEPRESSION
UTERINE CANCER	PREGNANCY COMPLICATIONS
BREAST CANCER	

eat too little of the right things. Mouthful by mouthful, they increase their vulnerability to diabetes, cardiovascular disease, osteoarthritis, breathing problems, some forms of cancer, and many other diseases, with too little nutritional food and too much high-fat, high-sodium, high-sugar, and refined-carbohydrate food. Of the nearly seven hundred thousand adult deaths every year in the United States, roughly three hundred thousand are attributable to unhealthy dietary habits and inactive lifestyles.[1,2]

Eighteen million people have type 2 diabetes.[3] Twenty million people have impaired glucose tolerance (prediabetes).[4] Seventeen million require ambulatory care for hypertension each year.[5] About a third of all Americans, 101 million, have cholesterol high enough to pose the risk of heart disease.[6]

Part of the problem is bad food—food with too much that leads to weight gain and disease and too little that leads to better health. According to another USDA study, the Healthy Eating Index, fewer than 10 percent of all Americans actually eat right. Greater than 16 percent eat really poorly. Those 48 million, plus a good number of the borderline eaters, are putting away way too much saturated fat, salt, sugar, and refined carbs. By eating these foods instead of plenty of fresh fruits, vegetables, and whole grains, they increase their vulnerability to disease.

The Inactivity Factor

The rest of the problem is too much food—an imbalance between calories in and calories out. We Americans are consuming too many calories, and we are burning fewer and fewer. Between 1973 and 2000, our per capita intake went up 716 calories per day. (In the United Kingdom, which was right behind us in this race to eat more, intake went up only 220 calories per day.) The average man eats approximately 2,700 calories a day.

That average man would have to play golf nine hours a day—without a golf cart—to burn all those calories. How often does that happen?

Instead, we are spending most of our time sitting, slumping, and sacked out—behind the wheel, at the office, and on the couch. Cave people and even preindustrial humans had to burn calories to get calories. All we have to do now is pass five bucks out the window at the drive-through.

Factor It All Together

To be fair, it is a mistake to expect a triangular graphic image to reshape America's eating habits and deliver vitality packaged in great physiques. Nevertheless, the USDA shouldered the challenge and went back to the drawing board. Clearly, either too few people were actually heeding the old-fashioned food pyramid's advice or something was missing from the message. The USDA nutritionists decided the pyramid failed in both categories. My Pyramid is the USDA's stab at making the message more persuasive . . . and more comprehensive. Together, irrefutable new facts and fresh ideas have turned the former pyramid on its side.

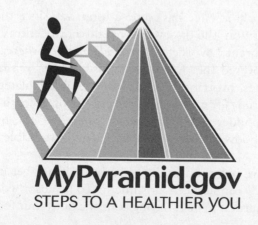

MyPyramid.gov
STEPS TO A HEALTHIER YOU

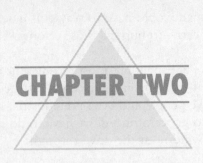

CHAPTER TWO

You Are What You Eat

What Is in Food?

You will learn that My Pyramid's recommendations are an important and helpful measure toward getting well. To understand *why*, let's look at what scientists have discovered over the last three hundred years—what food is, what it does, and how it does it.

Nutritional science has come a long way since the "first" news in nutrition: the discovery by eighteenth-century chemist Antoine-Laurent Lavoisier of *metabolism*. Soon thereafter, scientists discovered that food is composed of *macronutrients*—carbohydrates, proteins, and fats—and they calculated energy values (calories) for each. Then, during the nineteenth century, physicians pondered the process of *digestion*—the means by which the body converts food to useful, oxidizable components.

When we put food in our mouths, it is not yet in a form that the body can use as nourishment. To be absorbed into the blood and carried to cells throughout the body, our foods must

Metabolism

Food fuel supplies energy to the body through metabolism. *Metabolism is a chemical process through which living cells assimilate food. Catalyzed by hormones and enzymes, cells release energy in step-by-step chemical reactions. The energy yielded by one chemical reaction drives other reactions, all leading to oxidation and the gradual release of carbon dioxide, water, . . . and ultimately* energy, *the heat units that make us go. More simply, you can also think about your metabolism as the number of calories you are burning at any given moment.*

be changed into smaller molecules by digestion. Foods are broken down into the following components:

1. Energy-supplying compounds that make us go by delivering calories. These are the macronutrients:
   ▲ Carbohydrates
   ▲ Fats
   ▲ Protein
2. Building blocks that help us grow and regenerate cells:
   ▲ Protein
   ▲ Minerals
3. Catalysts that prompt chemical reactions to maintain health:
   ▲ Vitamins
   ▲ Trace elements
   ▲ Essential fatty acids

There is more to food than just energy supply, however. (This is something most Americans overlook, believing that as long as we are chewing, we will continue to go.) During the twentieth century, *micronutrients*—vitamins, minerals, trace elements, and essential fatty acids—took the spotlight. It turns out that our bodies need micronutrients to make metabolism efficient. Micronutrients also ensure the nutritional quality of the food, the difference between whether food makes you feel well or not—good fuel and bad fuel, if you will.

Carbohydrates are found in grain products (pasta, bread, rice, and baked goods), corn, potatoes and other vegetables, fruit, and sugar. They are made of thousands of glucose molecules. The digestive system breaks these molecules down into individual glucose molecules, which then enter the bloodstream. If not used immediately for energy, glucose is con-

Calories Are Only a Part of Food's Value

The macronutrients (carbohydrates, fats, and protein) deliver fuel in increments called calories. *These units of measure "pay" for certain amounts of energy expenditure. Calories are not the whole story, however. Yes, you can get more energy from a candy bar (about 300 calories) than you can from an apple (about 80 calories), but the candy bar may not provide the micronutrients (vitamins, minerals, trace elements, and essential fatty acids) your body requires to keep conditioned. The* metabolic pathways *that lead to food's absorption require interaction between nutrients and other dietary bioactives at the molecular level.*

verted to glycogen and stored in the liver and muscles. Once these reserves are filled, and calorie needs have been met, glucose is converted to fat and deposited in adipose (fatty) tissue.

Fats are found in butter, margarine, vegetable oils, sauces, salad dressings, all but nonfat milk products, baked goods, nuts, seeds, visibly on meat, and invisibly on fish and shellfish. Fat is the most concentrated of the energy-producing nutrients, so our bodies need relatively small amounts. Bile acids usher fat molecules through our blood. Fat consists of fatty acids attached to a substance called glycerol. If unused for energy, fat may be stored in the tissues for withdrawal when needed.

Protein is found in meat, poultry, fish, shellfish, nuts, seeds, legumes, grains, milk products, and eggs. Protein takes longer than carbohydrates and fats to digest, but the process is similar. Enzymes break down huge protein molecules into small molecules called *amino acids.* (More information on amino acids can be found under "The Meat and Beans Group" in Chapter 4.) These small molecules can be absorbed into the blood and delivered to every cell in order to build and repair body tissues.[7] Cell molecules rearrange amino acids into the proteins that the cells need. The body depends on protein for metabolism. Moreover, *hemoglobin,* the oxygen-carrying molecule of the blood, is built from protein.

Minerals and trace elements contain no calories (no energy); however, they are the basis of all matter on earth. They provide structural and functional support and assist the body in energy production. The body can utilize minerals, store them, or eliminate them. Since minerals sometimes compete with each other, it is best to feed your body a steady supply in the form of wholesome foods.

Vitamins are organic compounds essential to enhancement of the metabolism of amino acids, carbohydrates, and fats in living organisms. This means that even though vitamins do not impart energy (fuel) on their own, they are necessary to turn energy-providing foods into energy. Humans cannot synthesize vitamins and must obtain them from their food. Vitamins contribute to a variety of biochemical processes, such as nutrient absorption, immune system support, and DNA synthesis. Some vitamins are water soluble; others are fat soluble. Fats in the diet, in moderation, boost fat-soluble vitamin absorption. Water-soluble vitamins are not stored in the body; this increases the need to consume vitamin-rich produce and grains.[8]

Essential fatty acids are polyunsaturated fatty acids that, for the most part, our bodies cannot produce. Therefore, we must eat foods that contain linoleic, linolenic, and arachidonic acids (omega-3 and omega-6 fatty acids). They are important for normal growth, blood vessel and nerve support, maintaining healthy blood pressure, and lubricating skin and other tissues. Fats are digested mostly in the small intestine, helped along by bile secreted from the gallbladder.

Pulling the Food Components Together

The body functions best when all these components are supplied *in optimum quality and optimum proportions.* As far as quality is concerned, as you will learn later in this book, not all carbohydrates are equal. Not all proteins are good for you. Some fats may lead to disease. When it comes to proportion, about half our calories should be carbohydrates . . . but not just any carbohydrates—healthful complex carbohydrates. These are just examples.

The idea is to get the quality and proportions to meet nutrient needs. The *Recommended Daily Allowances,* known as RDAs (see pages 17–18), are the most recognized recommendations for nutrients. The RDAs average the amount of a nutrient that is needed for *most* people to stay healthy. They are different for children and adults, and for males and females.

The Dietary Reference Intakes—developed in response to increased knowledge about differences between genders, ages,

U.S. Recommended Daily Allowances (RDAs)

Compound	Units	Adult Males (25+ yrs.)	Adult Females (25+ yrs.)	Children (4-8 yrs.)	Infants (6-12 mos.)	Pregnant	Lactating*
Biotin	mcg	30†	30†	12†	6†	30†	35†
Calcium (Ca)	mg	1,200†	1,200†	800†	270†	1,000†	1,000†
Chloride (Cl)	mg	750	750	600	300	750	750
Chromium (Cr)	mcg	50–200	50–200	50–200	20–60	50–200	50–200
Copper (Cu)	mg	1.5–3	1.5–3	1–2	0.6–0.7	1.5–3	1.5–3
Fluoride (F)	mg	4†	3†	1†	0.5†	3†	3†
Folate	mcg	400†	400†	200†	80†	600†	500†
Iodine (I)	mcg	150	150	120	50	175	200
Iron (Fe)	mg	10	(25–50 yrs.) 15, (51+ yrs.) 10	10	10	30	15
Magnesium (Mg)	mg	420‡	320‡	130‡	75*	350–400‡	310–360‡
Manganese (Mn)	mg	2–5	2–5	2–3	0.6–1.0	2–5	2–5
Molybdenum (Mo)	mcg	75–250	75–250	50–150	20–40	75–250	75–250
Niacin	mg	16†	14‡	8‡	4†	18‡	17‡
Pantothenic	mg	5†	5†	3†	1.8†	6†	7†
Phosphorus (P)	mg	700‡	700‡	500‡	275†	700‡	700‡
Potassium (K)	mg	2,000	2,000	1,600	700	2,000	2,000
Protein	g	63	50	28	14	60	65
Selenium (Se)	mcg	70	55	30	15	65	75
Sodium (Na)	mg	500	500	400	200	500	500
Vitamin A	mcg RE†	1,000	800	700	375	800	1,300

U.S. Recommended Daily Allowances (RDAs) (continued)

Compound	Units	Adult Males (25+ yrs.)	Adult Females (25+ yrs.)	Children (4–8 yrs.)	Infants (6–12 mos.)	Pregnant	Lactating*
Vitamin B$_1$ (Thiamine)	mg	1.2‡	1.1‡	0.6‡	0.3†	1.4‡	1.5‡
Vitamin B$_2$ (Riboflavin)	mg	1.3‡	1.1‡	0.6‡	0.4†	1.4‡	1.6‡
Vitamin B$_6$ (Pyridoxine)	mg	1.7‡	1.5‡	0.6‡	0.3†	1.9‡	2.0‡
Vitamin B$_{12}$ (Cyanocobalamin)	mcg	2.4‡	2.4‡	1.2‡	0.5†	2.6‡	2.8‡
Vitamin C	mg	60	60	45	35	95	90
Vitamin D	mcg	(51–70 yrs.) 15† 10†, (71+ yrs.)	15† (51–70 yrs.)	15† (1–8 yrs.) 5†	5†	5†	5†
Vitamin E	mg alpha TE†	10	8	7	4	12	11
Vitamin K	mcg	80	65	30	10	65	65
Zinc (Zn)	mg	15	12	10	5	15	19

g = grams
mg = milligrams (0.001 g)
mcg = micrograms (0.000001 g)
IU = International Units
RE = Retinol Equivalent
Alpha TE = alpha Tocopherol Equivalent
*Generally the higher number was reported.
†AI (Adequate Intake) from the new Dietary Reference Intakes, National Academy of Sciences 1997: Calcium, Phosphorus, Magnesium, Vitamin D, and Fluoride. Values have changed from previous RDA.
‡RDA (Recommended Daily Allowance) from the new Dietary Reference Intakes, 1997: Calcium, Phosphorus, Magnesium, Vitamin D, and Fluoride. Values have changed from previous RDA.[9]

activity levels, genetic predispositions, and medical conditions—are a lot more complicated and comprehensive and may require professional translation to be put into use.

In the meantime, average Americans need a way to translate the DRIs into usable form by identifying amounts to consume from each food group and subgroup at a variety of energy levels. That is what My Pyramid recommendations are all about.

Why Is It So Hard to Eat Well to Feel Well?

Increased knowledge about how food works is not enough to cure us, though. Our bodies reflect what we put into them, what we do, and where and how we live.

Food is fuel. Not all automobile fuel is the same; likewise, there are dramatic differences between foods. There are also differences in how they are absorbed and utilized from person to person. As with a car, if you tank up on inferior fuel by eating "empty," or poor-quality, calories, your body will not perform well. It may even "misfire" by becoming stressed, overweight, and diseased. This is because food is composed of chemicals, and these chemicals prompt chemical reactions in our system, good or bad. Knowing this, it is prudent to aim for the best chemistry possible. Yet our inability to get the most out of our food sources is a growing problem in the United States for several reasons.

Food Has Changed

In simpler times, before the mass commercialization of food products, people lived and ate closer to food sources. They ate whole foods. They knew their grocers, and their grocers knew their vendors and farmers. There was more rich topsoil. There was less pollution. There were fewer chemical additives. Processed food, in the form we know today, did not exist.

In the drive to fill commercial demand at the least possible cost and increase shelf life and visual appeal, the quality of some foods deteriorates. Even though great advances have occurred in food cultivation, food suppliers today are delivering foods that were raised far from most people's lives and often harvested weeks and sometimes months in advance of being sold. In many cases, their ultimate form is very different from that of the original food resources that contribute to their composition. We know that food is not just hatched at the grocer's, but we cannot know the conditions under which it originated on farms and ranches and in the sea. Many of America's foods come from abroad, where strict environmental rules may not apply. Since we cannot measure how the produce is cultivated or what the animals eat, we cannot know how nutritious it actually is unless it is packaged and labeled, as processed food is. Even then, the labels actually tell us very little. As consumers, we must now consider that just because one tomato is big and red, this does not mean it is as healthful as some other tomato.

Imported Produce

Imported fruits and vegetables make up some 40 percent of the produce consumed in this country.[10] *This statistic reminds us how difficult it is to know the conditions under which foods are cultivated and how many nutrients they still contain when they get here.*

The market is flooded with convenience foods that are not necessarily as good for us as whole fresh foods. Not always, but generally, the more removed a food is from its original state, the more it loses nutritional value. Lettuce harvested last week does not supply as many nutrients as that picked today. Removing outer leaves and peels from produce removes some nutrients.[11] Inexpensive, processed ingredients in some packaged and fast food may have much-reduced value.

To decrease or eliminate harmful bacteria, the Food and Drug Administration (FDA) approves irradiation of meat and poultry and allows its use for fresh fruits, vegetables, and spices. The agency says that the process is safe and effective. Irradiation reduces spoilage bacteria, insects, and parasites, and in certain fruits and vegetables it inhibits sprouting and delays ripening. For example, irradiated strawberries stay unspoiled up to three weeks, versus three to five days for untreated berries. Some believe that, in addition to keeping food on the market long after it has been harvested, thereby decreasing its nutritional value when it is consumed, food irradiation masks what may be unsanitary conditions in food processing plants.

What about the chemicals used in preparing foods for sale to consumers? Yes, some go into the finished product and are thus on the labels. Those are FDA-approved. Others are not listed because they are used only in cultivation and processing. Chemicals used in pesticides and fungicides and petroleum-based chemicals used in hydrogenating oils are two examples. It is good to remember, when eyeing a label loaded with unrecognizable ingredients, that our bodies evolved to eat *real food*, not stuff cooked up in a laboratory.

There is also controversy surrounding high-tech genetic engineering. Unlike the European Union, which adopted the Biosafety Protocol to protect consumers who are opposed to genetically modified organisms (GMOs), U.S. agribusinesses have embraced genetically engineered corn and other crops—particularly corn, canola (rapeseed), and soybeans. As a result, unless labels specifically state that these contents have *not* been genetically engineered, there is a strong likelihood that they have been. The jury is still out on whether GMOs are, to any degree, bad for us.

Then there is junk food. High-fat, high-cholesterol, and high-sugar foods are not just empty; they are injurious. They contribute to health problems and weight problems. The problem is that too many people equate meals built of junk food with fuel. The mistake may mean not just added weight; chemical reactions that result from eating junk food may activate disease-causing genes or disable health maintenance genes. The new pyramid is a means of awakening consumers to these issues.

Eating Has Changed

At the same time, civilization is increasingly busy. How many men and women can afford to spend their time at home, planning and making nutritious meals? Ever fewer people go to work or school carrying home-prepared lunches. Families rely on packaged and processed food, heat-and-eat food, fast food, and restaurants when they have the money. Forty-six percent of all Americans eat out every day, and one-third of them eat calorie-rich and nutrient-poor fast food.[12] Clearly, *food consumption patterns* are being transformed—and not necessarily in good directions.

Even when we do eat at home, we tend to eat prepared or partially prepared food. Only about a third of home-cooked meals are made from scratch.[13] When shopping, consumers try to compensate by choosing convenience foods with "no fat" or "low fat" on the label, disregarding the products' other ingredients. Preservatives, sodium (salt), and synthetic nutrients do not re-create nature. As a result, we may be getting fewer and fewer of the nutrients we sorely need. We are putting away increasing volumes of processed food, yet our bodies remain genetically programmed to thrive on the whole foods of our ancestors.

The Environment Has Changed

Pollution now taxes our systems more than ever before. Rising populations, industrialization, and development are leading to more pollution in our air, soil, and water. Allergens proliferate. Sources of pollution are not just "out there." They may be in our homes, our workplaces, our clothes, our food, and our bodies. A National Health and Nutrition Survey looked for 116 environmental chemicals in the civilian U.S. population and found them all.[14] Pollution destabilizes our well-being by creating *free radicals* within us. In our bodies, free radicals precipitate chain reactions that disrupt one cell after another (more about this in Chapter 4). The proliferation of free radicals uses up nutrients. This rising demand is occurring at the same time that dietary intake is depreciating.

Lifestyles Have Changed

These are increasingly stressful times. Every time you feel worried, sad, or mad, your body reacts chemically. Like pollution, anxiety destabilizes our systems by creating free radicals. Stress uses up extra nutrients and makes existing nutrients more difficult to assimilate. In addition, stress often leads to overeating—and overeating the wrong foods. Anxious, upset people do not usually reach for carrot sticks; they reach for chocolate, chips, and/or alcohol.

Meanwhile, against a backdrop of anxiety, Americans are becoming more inert and less physically active. According to the Centers for Disease Control, 25 percent of adults are entirely inactive, getting no exercise at all. Another 45 percent do not engage in regular activity. This is *half* the number of those who exercised fifteen years ago. Increasingly, urbanized settings work against regular outdoor activities. Dense traffic, crime, and lack of open space restrain populations—either at home, at

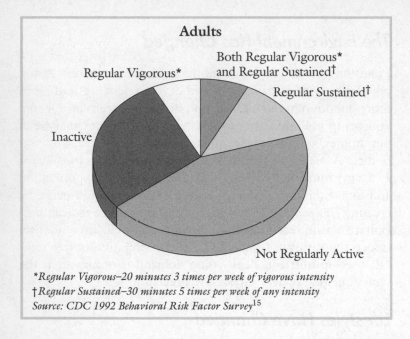

Adults

Both Regular Vigorous*
and Regular Sustained†

Regular Vigorous*

Regular Sustained†

Inactive

Not Regularly Active

*Regular Vigorous–20 minutes 3 times per week of vigorous intensity
†Regular Sustained–30 minutes 5 times per week of any intensity
Source: CDC 1992 Behavioral Risk Factor Survey[15]

work, or in the car—all too often with less-nutritious snack food
as their pal.

Depression and anxiety can be another disincentive for exercise. According to the October 22, 2004 issue of *Morbidity
and Mortality Weekly Report,* published by the U.S. Centers for
Disease Control and Prevention, the prevalence of U.S. adults
with "frequent mental distress" increased from 8.4 percent to
10.1 percent of the population between 1993 and 2001.[16] Instead of exercising to feel better, many people who suffer from
depression simply take medicine. While physical activity decreased, sales of antidepressants rose 800 percent during the
1990s.[17]

Whether it's because people are busy, locked into the con-
crete jungle, or too blue to move, their lack of exercise tends to
lead to weight gain. Sedentary lifestyles can also lead to disease.
Both weight gain and disease are related to what and how people eat. No wonder the 1992 Food Pyramid came up wanting.

The proof that poor food, poor eating habits, a poor environment, and poor lifestyles are dangerous is in America's horrendous health statistics. We are what we eat, and we are not well. We are improperly fueled. If we were cars instead of humans, we'd be sputtering, backfiring, breaking down, and abandoned on the roadsides. All four factors underscore why, as an overweight, diseased population, we need the fresh start My Pyramid provides and the better fuel it recommends.

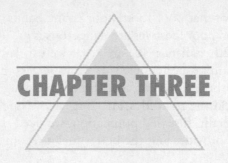

CHAPTER THREE

Pyramid Power Improves Your Health and Weight

Reinventing the Pyramid

As is evident from the data in Chapter 1 and the shifts described in Chapter 2, the reasons for revamping the pyramid were very compelling. The old pyramid was outdated, and consumers did not follow its advice. Getting Americans to get serious about their health might take a figurative slap in the face or kick in the behind.

The U.S. Department of Agriculture (USDA) went to work, with the goal of incorporating the latest science and making *not a diet*, but a set of nutritional and educational tools. They aimed for a "food guidance system" that was much more motivating than the old food pyramid. The result, My Pyramid, took four years and $2.4 million.

Steps to Creating the Steps

My Pyramid: Steps to a Healthier You is a food guidance system. To create it, the USDA

1. Assessed the new data on nutritional content of foods

2. Factored in food intake patterns

3. Developed consumer-friendly advice to foster behavioral changes

4. Included focused messages

5. Incorporated individualized educational tools

6. Tailored information to a multitude of personal needs

7. Designed a new symbol, slogan, and Web-based educational materials

8. Solicited public comment

9. Tested on consumers and revised

As a basis for the science, the USDA used several sources. The National Academy of Sciences' Institute of Medicine replaced the former Recommended Daily Allowances (RDAs) with the much more complicated Dietary Reference Intakes (DRIs). *The Dietary Guidelines for Americans,* the cornerstone of federal nutrition policy created by the USDA and the U.S. Department of Health and Human Services, was updated for release in 2005. And the USDA's Agricultural Research Service released new data on the nutritional content of foods and food consumption patterns.

These sources and others were distilled, then developed into the sought-after food guidance system to replace the original pyramid. The USDA sent the proposed plan out for public review and comment in July 2004. Comments helped refine the food guidance system.

Meanwhile, the "tools" experts went to work to design specific, consumer-friendly advice designed to encourage behavioral changes. The USDA hired Porter Novelli International, a public relations firm that has other health and food clients, to create a new logo and the "Steps to a Healthier You" slogan. In addition to this, the USDA developed educational materials and—capitalizing on Americans' love affair with electronics—an interactive website.

The results, delivering on the promise to offer Americans comprehensive guidance on how to eat a nutritious diet and maintain a healthy weight, were released April 19, 2005.

Anatomy of the My Pyramid Logo

Even though people did not necessarily follow the old horizontal pyramid's advice, the message of its labeled stack of food groups was clear: Eat more foods from the wide spaces lower on the pyramid and fewer foods from the narrow spaces near the top. Because the new pyramid logo does not have food labels for easy recognition, it is more complicated to understand and impossible without the website, instructional materials, or printed media such as this book. To be fair, how-

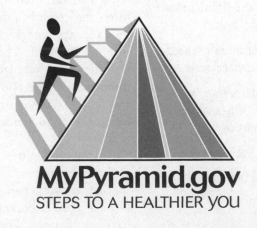

ever, a lot of logos do not make sense until you know what they represent.

Start with the objective behind the My Pyramid symbol: *to remind consumers to make healthy food choices and be active every day*. The icon components, as well as their size, shape, and configuration, add up to the best of what science has to offer, yet they need some explaining.

Variation is symbolized by the six different-colored vertical bands (displayed here in black-and-white, but in color on the cover of this book and on the website), representing *Grains, Vegetables, Fruits, Milk, Meat and Beans,* and *Oils* in a rainbow of foods. Selections from all groups are needed each day for good health.

Moderation is represented by the narrowing of each food group from bottom to top. The wider base indicates foods with little or no solid fats or added sugars. Select these more often. The narrower top area indicates foods containing more solid fats and added sugars. If you exercise, you can eat more of these foods without gaining weight or hurting your health.

Proportionality is shown by the different widths of the food group bands. The widths suggest how much food a person should choose from each group. These are not exact; rather, they are just a general guide.

Physical activity, a key addition to the USDA's wellness message, is represented by the steps and the person climbing them. The steps send another message, too. Developing the discipline and habits to change one's dietary and physical regime takes time. The logo—like the slogan "Steps to a Healthier You"—encourages users to make changes, one step at a time.

Personalization and *gradual improvement* are shown by the person on the steps, the slogan "Steps to a Healthier You," the website (www.mypyramid.gov), and, indeed, this book. All encourage you to modify portions based on your age, gender, and activity level.

The Interactive Website

The My Pyramid: Steps to a Healthier You website invites greater conformance by making food tracking like a computer game. It has a wealth of information, as long as you have the stamina to keep clicking. Almost everything on the site links to more information. It makes you work harder (and perhaps even burn more calories) to figure out whether what you are eating is good for you. Using the advice can help you

▲ Make smart choices from every food group

▲ Find your balance between food and physical activity

▲ Get the most nutrition out of your calories

▲ Craft and test a dietary regime that works for you

You can get the same benefits from this book. However, whereas the website calibrates calorie burning to calorie intake, if you are using the book, you have to do your own math.

One Size Doesn't Fit All

Unlike the previous pyramid, My Pyramid demonstrates differences between foods in the same category . . . and between humans.

Differences within Food Categories

The My Pyramid food category bands start out wider at the bottom and get thinner as they taper to the top. This reminds us that not all foods are created equal, even within a healthy food group like fruit. Take, for instance, apples and apple pie. Whereas a fresh apple would be at the wide part of the fruit category with foods that have stronger nutritional content, apple pie would be at the thinner part. The less fat and added sugar a food item has, the closer it is to the wholesome base of the pyramid. The more nutrients is has, by virtue of its freshness and preparation, the closer it is to the wholesome base of the pyramid. The more our dietary choices conform to the base of the pyramid, the better.

Nutritional Requirement Differences between People

Before, following the old Food Pyramid, food recommendations did not shift much, except in the Grain Group. Whether you were a man, a woman, or a child, whether you were an athlete or an invalid, whether you were a newborn or a twenty-year-old, the old pyramid still seemed to guide you to eat the same proportions of fruits, milk products, vegetables, and fruit.

By contrast, My Pyramid: Steps to a Healthier You accommodates different genders, ages, and activity levels. It is more personalized. It does not immediately provide the specific food group and portion information of the previous pyramid. However, for a quick estimate of what and how much you need to eat, you can simply enter your age, sex, and activity level in the My Pyramid Plan box on the website.

A page immediately pops up telling you how many servings of each food group you need to eat daily to meet the guidelines. The advice is straightforward: A forty-five-year-old man who exercises between thirty and sixty minutes a day should consume 2,200 calories daily. Those calories should come from 9 ounces of grains (half of them whole grains), 3.5 cups of vegetables, 2 cups of fruit, 3 cups of milk products, 6.5 ounces of protein (lean meat, poultry, fish, nuts, eggs, or beans), and 8 teaspoons of healthful oil (margarine, olive oil, nuts, avocados). By contrast, a sixty-two-year-old sedentary woman should eat 1,600 calories daily from 5 ounces of grains (half of them whole grains); 2 cups of vegetables, 1½ cups of fruit; 3 cups of milk products, 5 ounces of protein, and 5 teaspoons of healthful oil.

You can also choose the foods and amounts that are right for you by using this book.

The website shows six colored food-group segments: orange for grains, green for vegetables, red for fruit, yellow for healthful oils, blue for milk, and purple for lean meat, poultry, seafood, beans, and eggs. Clicking on each one directs you into that specific food group and presents a cornucopia of information on why each food group is vitally important to your health and weight. The website also tells you how much of an individual food constitutes a portion.

Chapter 4 of this book also gives you this food group information.

The new stairway image on the pyramid reminds users to be more active. A few clicks on Physical Activity and you will find out how many calories various activities burn (based on a 154-pound man), read tips for incorporating more physical activity into your life, and learn the health benefits of exercise.

Chapter 6 of this book covers these same physical activity topics.

The website includes an online dietary intake and physical activity assessment tool called My Pyramid Tracker (http://mypyramidtracker.gov/), which will track up to a year's worth of food and exercise records, then create graphs that compare results to the *Dietary Guidelines*. It can help you improve your eating and exercise habits and maintain your weight or guide you toward reaching a healthier weight.

After you input information about the food you eat and the

physical activities you do in any given day, My Pyramid Tracker gives feedback in the form of emoticons.

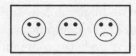

These tell you whether or not you have eaten prudently, according to the *Dietary Guidelines for Americans, 2005.* My Pyramid Tracker also reports on your nutrient intake and tells you whether you have had too much solid fat or added sugar.

The physical activity meter calibrates your caloric expenditures from activity and lets you know whether they are good or bad. As with the food intake feature, inputting all the data takes some time. After the system has recorded all your eating and activities for the day, its Energy Balance feature automatically calculates your energy balance by subtracting the energy you expend on physical activity from your food calories/energy intake. Energy Balance tells you whether what you are eating and doing will result in weight gain, weight loss, or weight stability.

Most people—even those who think they eat and exercise well—are startled to discover where their shortcomings lie. If you have access to a computer, it is a good idea to take the time to input this food and exercise data for a few days using My Pyramid Tracker—just to see where you are off track and by how much.

Not All the Buzz about My Pyramid Is Positive

The main drawback to using My Pyramid is how long it takes. The interactive website is informative, but it is as time-consuming to navigate as a holiday exodus from a big city at rush hour. Moreover, not everyone has access to a computer. Some people—especially those who already struggle to get some nutrition from the subquality foods that less-affluent people tend to buy and who might already suffer from diet-related illnesses—may have neither a computer nor the time to use the website. Even those who do have computers may not have time to input everything they eat each day.

A further drawback is that it is difficult to figure out how much food constitutes a portion without using the website's equivalency charts. Unless you are a nutrition professional, you really need the charts to tell you what quantity of any food is sufficient to meet nutritional requirements.

Furthermore, some scientists and nutritionists have taken exception to the USDA's evident support for the dairy and meat industries, as reflected in the recommendations for the Milk and Meat and Beans food groups. Nor does it disserve traditional agribusiness by coming out in favor of organic products; in fact, there are only nine references to organic products on the vast website. In a market increasingly concerned about genetically modified organisms, hormone additives, chemical fertilizers, pesticides, and herbicides, this seems a major shortfall. My Pyramid does provide information on lactose intolerance and vegetarianism, as well as other means of recognizing the value of nondairy, nonanimal foods, which are potentially helpful to nearly everyone and further the goal of improving health and reducing susceptibility to chronic diseases through diet.

This book is designed to make the My Pyramid recommendations more usable for everyone all the time. It cannot give you quick feedback on what you ate and the physical activities you performed, as My Pyramid Tracker does, nor does it offer the Energy Balance feature. However, this book does give you enough information to calculate this information for yourself. Best of all, unlike the website, you can take the book with you to restaurants and the grocery store and use it in the kitchen while you cook.

How Much Must You Change Your Diet?

The program My Pyramid recommends does not seem that difficult. Most people eat from the six food groups already. As you will read in Chapter 4, the problem arises with the *selections* from the food groups and the *proportions* that are recommended. The traditional burger is a good example. It supplies everything except something from the fruit group. But to "get with the program," the bun would have to be at least half whole-grain, the lettuce and tomato would have to be very fresh and abundant, the mayo would have to be made with nonhydrogenated vegetable oil, and the meat would have to be very lean and the patty a lot smaller than usual.

The following graphs show how much, on average, most Americans would need to change what they eat to meet My Pyramid recommendations. The bars above the zero line represent recommended *increases* in food group consumption, while the bars below the line represent recommended *decreases*.

According to the first chart, it looks as if we do not have to change that much—except for eating half again as many vegetables, twice as many fruits, and a good bit more from the milk group (unless you are lactose-intolerant, in which case you must eat more vegetables and meat or beans). But study the second chart for a minute. It clearly shows that french fries and baked potatoes are not enough to meet the vegetable allotment. For a start, we should be eating between two and three times as many leafy greens and three times as many whole grains. These are pretty demanding changes.

The chart was created from the USDA Food Guide in comparison to National Health and Nutrition Examination Survey 2001–2002 consumption data. Increases in the amounts recommended for some food groups are offset by decreases in the amounts of solid fats (i.e., saturated and trans

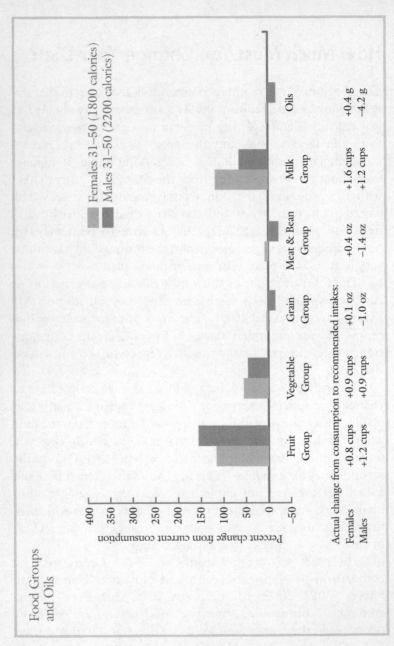

Food Groups
and Oils

Percent change from current consumption

- Females 31–50 (1800 calories)
- Males 31–50 (2200 calories)

	Fruit Group	Vegetable Group	Grain Group	Meat & Bean Group	Milk Group	Oils
Actual change from consumption to recommended intakes:						
Females	+0.8 cups	+0.9 cups	+0.1 oz	+0.4 oz	+1.6 cups	+0.4 g
Males	+1.2 cups	+0.9 cups	–1.0 oz	–1.4 oz	+1.2 cups	–4.2 g

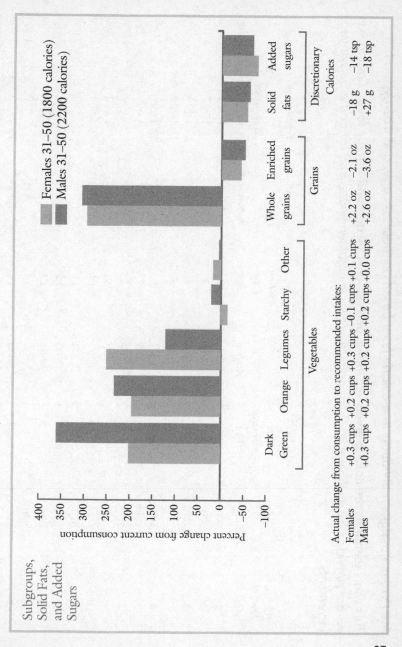

Subgroups, Solid Fats, and Added Sugars

Females 31–50 (1800 calories)
Males 31–50 (2200 calories)

Percent change from current consumption

400
350
300
250
200
150
100
50
0
-50
-100

Dark Green   Orange   Legumes   Starchy   Other

Vegetables

Whole grains   Enriched grains

Grains

Solid fats   Added sugars

Discretionary Calories

Actual change from consumption to recommended intakes:

	Dark Green	Orange	Legumes	Starchy	Other	Whole grains	Enriched grains	Solid fats	Added sugars
Females	+0.3 cups	+0.2 cups	+0.3 cups	–0.1 cups	+0.1 cups	+2.2 oz	–2.1 oz	–18 g	–14 tsp
Males	+0.3 cups	+0.2 cups	+0.2 cups	+0.2 cups	+0.0 cups	+2.6 oz	–3.6 oz	+27 g	–18 tsp

Daily Calorie Levels

My Pyramid assigns individuals to a calorie level based on their sex, age, and activity level.

This chart identifies the calorie levels for males and females by age and activity level. Calorie levels are provided for each year of childhood, from two to eighteen years, and for adults in five-year increments.

Activity Level Age	Males Sedentary*	Males Moderately active*	Males Active*	Females Sedentary*	Females Moderately active*	Females Active*
2	1,000	1,000	1,000	1,000	1,000	1,000
3	1,000	1,400	1,400	1,000	1,200	1,400
4	1,200	1,400	1,600	1,200	1,400	1,400
5	1,200	1,400	1,600	1,200	1,400	1,600
6	1,400	1,600	1,800	1,200	1,400	1,600
7	1,400	1,600	1,800	1,200	1,600	1,800
8	1,400	1,600	2,000	1,400	1,600	1,800
9	1,600	1,800	2,000	1,400	1,600	1,800
10	1,600	1,800	2,200	1,400	1,800	2,000
11	1,800	2,000	2,200	1,600	1,800	2,000
12	1,800	2,200	2,400	1,600	2,000	2,200
13	2,000	2,200	2,600	1,600	2,000	2,200
14	2,000	2,400	2,800	1,800	2,000	2,400
15	2,200	2,600	3,000	1,800	2,000	2,400
16	2,400	2,800	3,200	1,800	2,000	2,400
17	2,400	2,800	3,200	1,800	2,000	2,400

Daily Calorie Levels (continued)

Activity Level Age	Males			Females		
	Sedentary*	Moderately active*	Active*	Sedentary*	Moderately active*	Active*
18	2,400	2,800	3,200	1,800	2,000	2,400
19–20	2,600	2,800	3,000	2,000	2,200	2,400
21–25	2,400	2,800	3,000	2,000	2,200	2,400
26–30	2,400	2,600	3,000	1,800	2,000	2,400
31–35	2,400	2,600	3,000	1,800	2,000	2,200
36–40	2,400	2,600	2,800	1,800	2,000	2,200
41–45	2,200	2,600	2,800	1,800	2,000	2,200
46–50	2,200	2,400	2,800	1,800	2,000	2,200
51–55	2,200	2,400	2,800	1,600	1,800	2,200
56–60	2,200	2,400	2,600	1,600	1,800	2,200
61–65	2,000	2,400	2,600	1,600	1,800	2,000
66–70	2,000	2,200	2,600	1,600	1,800	2,000
71–75	2,000	2,200	2,600	1,600	1,800	2,000
76 and up	2,000	2,200	2,400	1,600	1,800	2,000

*Calorie levels are based on the Estimated Energy Requirements (EER) and activity levels from the Institute of Medicine Dietary Reference Intakes Macronutrients Report, 2002.

Sedentary = less than thirty minutes a day of moderate physical activity in addition to daily activities.

Moderately active = at least thirty minutes up to sixty minutes a day of moderate physical activity in addition to daily activities.

Active = Sixty or more minutes a day of moderate physical activity in addition to daily activities.

MyPyramid.gov
STEPS TO A HEALTHIER YOU

MyPyramid Worksheet

Check how you did today and set a goal to aim for tomorrow

Write in Your Choices for Today	Food Group	Tip	Goal From _____ _____ total calories.	List each food choice in its food group*	Estimate Your Total
	GRAINS	Make at least half your grains whole grains	**ounce equivalents** (1 ounce equivalent is about 1 slice bread, 1 cup dry cereal, or ½ cup cooked rice, pasta, or cereal)		_____ ounce equivalents
	VEGETABLES	Try to have vegetables from several subgroups each day	_____ **cups** Subgroups: Dark Green, Orange, Starchy, Dry Beans and Peas, Other Veggies		_____ cups
	FRUITS	Make most choices fruit, not juice	_____ **cups**		_____ cups
	MILK	Choose fat-free or low fat most often	_____ **cups** (1 ½ ounces cheese = 1 cup milk)		_____ cups
	MEAT & BEANS	Choose lean meat and poultry. Vary your choices—more fish, beans, peas, nuts, and seeds	_____ **ounce equivalents** (1 ounce equivalent is 1 ounce meat, poultry, or fish, 1 egg, 1 T. peanut butter, ½ ounce nuts, or ¼ cup dry beans)		_____ ounce equivalents
	PHYSICAL ACTIVITY	Build more physical activity into your daily routine at home and work.	At least 30 minutes of moderate to vigorous activity a day, 10 minutes or more at a time.	*Some foods don't fit into any group. These "extras" may be mainly fat or sugar— limit your intake of these.	_____ minutes

How did you do today? ☐ Great   ☐ So-So   ☐ Not so Great

My food goal for tomorrow is: _____

My activity goal for tomorrow is: _____

40

MyPyramid.gov
STEPS TO A HEALTHIER YOU

MyPyramid Worksheet

Check how you did today and set a goal to aim for tomorrow

Write in Your Choices for Today	Food Group	Tip	Goal From _____ total calories.	List each food choice in its food group*	Estimate Your Total
	GRAINS	Make at least half your grains whole grains	**ounce equivalents** (1 ounce equivalent is about 1 slice bread, 1 cup dry cereal, or ½ cup cooked rice, pasta, or cereal)		_____ ounce equivalents
	VEGETABLES	Try to have vegetables from several subgroups each day	**cups** Subgroups: Dark Green, Orange, Starchy, Dry Beans and Peas, Other Veggies		_____ cups
	FRUITS	Make most choices fruit, not juice	— **cups**		_____ cups
	MILK	Choose fat-free or low fat most often	— **cups** (1 ½ ounces cheese = 1 cup milk)		_____ cups
	MEAT & BEANS	Choose lean meat and poultry. Vary your choices—more fish, beans, peas, nuts, and seeds	**ounce equivalents** (1 ounce equivalent is 1 ounce meat, poultry, or fish, 1 egg, 1 T. peanut butter, ½ ounce nuts, or ¼ cup dry beans)		_____ ounce equivalents
	PHYSICAL ACTIVITY	Build more physical activity into your daily routine at home and work.	At least 30 minutes of moderate to vigorous activity a day, 10 minutes or more at a time.	*Some foods don't fit into any group. These "extras" may be mainly fat or sugar—limit your intake of these.	_____ minutes

How did you do today? ☐ Great ☐ So-So ☐ Not so Great

My food goal for tomorrow is: _____

My activity goal for tomorrow is: _____

41

fats) and added sugars, so that total calorie intake is at the recommended level. For more information about the process,
summary data, and the resources used by the Advisory
Committee, see the 2005 Dietary Guidelines Advisory Committee Report (2005 DGAC Report) at www.health.gov/
dietaryguidelines.

Remember, these are averages and they may not correspond to the way you eat. The changes will make more sense as
you read Chapter 4, which will help you understand why such
changes may be critical and how you can incorporate them into
your own diet.

Like any "how-to" program, My Pyramid tells you what to
do, but it can't control your diet for you—the real work is still
up to you. This book will help you do the work, not just when
you are sitting at your computer using www.mypyramid.gov,
but *anywhere*. The chapters that follow will rev you up and inspire you with a can-do attitude.

Getting Ready to Record
Your Nutritional Progress

The My Pyramid website allows you to create an individualized
worksheet. Or you can create one of your own. Find your gender and age on the Daily Calorie Level chart on pages 38–39.
Then circle the calorie allotment that corresponds to your activity level.

Now, on the following food group chart, circle the column
of food group quantities that corresponds to your calorie allotment. For instance, if you are an active teenage boy or an adult
high-activity athlete, you might burn 3,200 calories a day. You
would circle the last column on the right.

On the My Pyramid Worksheet, insert your daily calorie allotment into the blank at the top of the Goal column. Then in-

Daily Amount of Food from Each Group

Calorie Level	1,000	1,200	1,400	1,600	1,800	2,000	2,200	2,400	2,600	2,800	3,000	3,200
Fruits	1 cup	1 cup	1.5 cups	1.5 cups	1.5 cups	2 cups	2 cups	2 cups	2 cups	2.5 cups	2.5 cups	2.5 cups
Vegetables	1 cup	1.5 cups	1.5 cups	2 cups	2.5 cups	2.5 cups	3 cups	3 cups	3.5 cups	3.5 cups	4 cups	4 cups
Grains	3 oz-eq	4 oz-eq	5 oz-eq	5 oz-eq	6 oz-eq	6 oz-eq	7 oz-eq	8 oz-eq	9 oz-eq	10 oz-eq	10 oz-eq	10 oz-eq
Meat and Beans	2 oz-eq	3 oz-eq	4 oz-eq	5 oz-eq	5 oz-eq	5.5 oz-eq	6 oz-eq	6.5 oz-eq	6.5 oz-eq	7 oz-eq	7 oz-eq	7 oz-eq
Milk	2 cups	2 cups	2 cups	3 cups	3 cups	3 cups	3 cups	3 cups	3 cups	3 cups	3 cups	3 cups
Oils	3 tsp	4 tsp	4 tsp	5 tsp	5 tsp	6 tsp	6 tsp	7 tsp	8 tsp	8 tsp	10 tsp	11 tsp
Discretionary calorie allowance	165	171	171	132	195	267	290	362	410	426	512	648

sert the recommended daily quantities from each food group in the table on page 43 in the blanks in the Goal column. For example, if you are a very active thirty-seven-year-old woman, your goals should be 7 ounce equivalents of grains, 3 cups of vegetables, 2 cups of fruits, 3 cups of milk products, 6 ounce equivalents of meat or beans, 6 teaspoons of oil, and 290 discretionary calories, all adding up to 2,200 calories.

Once you have filled in the blanks, copy a few of these sheets to use for coming days. Discipline yourself to fill them out and see whether you can improve your nutritional and exercise habits. Copy and post the worksheet on your refrigerator or carry it in your bag as a reference and to record what you eat.

CHAPTER FOUR

Taking Stock of Your Food Choices

Each of My Pyramid's six food groups plays a strong dietary role, both metabolically and nutritionally. Generally, people thrive on more of some categories and less of others—more grains than meats, more vegetables than oil, and so forth. Therefore, each food group appears as a different size on the My Pyramid symbol, representing the recommended portions of each. Prioritizing them as proposed by My Pyramid leads to vitality, decreases vulnerability to disease, and staves off hunger pangs. In addition, it helps you achieve your ideal weight. Eating as suggested can also afford you extra "discretionary" calories for those "sinful" foods you might crave.

The following pages take you through the six food groups, one at a time, explaining what they are, why they are important, and how you can make sure you get enough from each. The background information provided should dispel confusion about the My Pyramid program, and the charts will help you recognize how much of various foods counts as a serving.

The Grain Group

My Pyramid Directive: Consume three or more portions (1-ounce equivalents) of *whole-grain* products per day. Toddlers require only one and a half portions of whole-grain products, a requirement that grows as they mature. Additional recommended grains, within the allotment for your gender, age, and activity level, should come from enriched or whole-grain products. In total, at least half the grains should be whole grains.

What Is the Grain Group?

The large orange segment on the left side of the My Pyramid graphic represents the Grain Group, the foundation of everyone's diet. This priority is consistent with the previous Food Pyramid. Grain is still the food category from which we should eat the most servings—it is the "staff of life." However, that does not mean doughnuts as usual. It means prioritizing *unrefined complex carbohydrates* and *whole grains,* and holding back on the refined grains. Therefore, My Pyramid divides grains into two subgroups—*whole* and *refined*—and suggests that we make at least half our grain portions whole-grain foods.

First, let's distinguish between whole grains and refined grains.

Anatomy of a Grain

BRAN + GERM + ENDOSPERM = KERNEL

What Is a Whole-Grain Food?

We all know grains as bread, cereal, pasta, and rice, but few make the distinction between whole and refined grains. Whole grains include the bran, germ, and endosperm in relatively the same proportions as they were before the grain was crushed, cracked, or flaked. Beware: Wheat flour, enriched flour, and degerminated cornmeal are not whole grains. Foods with added bran are not whole grains. Foods labeled with the words *multigrain, stone-ground, 100 percent wheat, cracked wheat, seven-grain,* or *bran* do not necessarily indicate whole-grain products. Looking for breads and cereals that are browner or crunchier is not enough.

Whole-Grain Foods

WHOLE-WHEAT FLOUR

BULGUR (CRACKED WHEAT)

OATMEAL

WHOLE-GRAIN CORNMEAL

BROWN RICE

WILD RICE

AMARANTH

MILLET

QUINOA

SORGHUM

TRITICALE

POPCORN

WHOLE-WHEAT CEREAL FLAKES

MUESLI

WHOLE-GRAIN OR PEARL BARLEY

WHOLE RYE

WHOLE-WHEAT BREAD, BUNS, AND ROLLS

(continued)

WHOLE-WHEAT
  CRACKERS AND
  PRETZELS

WHOLE-WHEAT PASTA

BROWN-RICE PASTA

QUINOA PASTA

WHOLE-WHEAT
  TORTILLAS

WHOLE-MEAL
  (BRITISH WORD FOR
  WHOLE-WHEAT)

Note:

1. *Bran is not a whole grain but only the hull of the kernel. Though it supplies fiber, it does not supply vitamins and minerals because it is not technically digestible.*

2. *Whether whole-grain products are prepared traditionally or are labeled "quick" or "instant," they are still whole-grain foods.*

3. *Foods that contain primarily whole grains—such as muesli—count as whole-grain foods.*

What Is a Refined Grain?

When a grain is refined, most of the bran and some of the germ are eliminated, taking the dietary fiber, vitamins, minerals, and other useful nutrients such as lignans, phytoestrogens, phenolic compounds, and phytic acid with them. Refined grains have a finer texture and longer shelf life. Today, most refined grains are *enriched*. This means they are fortified with iron and B vitamins (folic acid, thiamin, riboflavin, and niacin). The fiber, however, is not replaced in enriched refined grains, unless bran is added.

Foods Made from
Refined Grains

CORN BREAD

CORN TORTILLAS,
　　UNLESS "WHOLE" IS
　　SPECIFIED

FLOUR TORTILLAS

COUSCOUS

CRACKERS AND
　　PRETZELS, UNLESS
　　THEY ARE WHOLE
　　WHEAT

GRITS

NOODLES AND PASTA,
　　UNLESS THEY ARE
　　WHOLE WHEAT

CORNFLAKES

WHITE BREAD, BUNS,
　　AND ROLLS

WHITE RICE

Note: Check the label. Some of these products are available in whole-grain versions.

Comparison of Nutrients: Whole-Grain Wheat Flour versus Enriched, Bleached, White, All-Purpose Flour

You can see from the following comparison chart why the USDA puts such a strong emphasis on whole grains. Most vitamins and minerals occur in much higher concentrations in whole-wheat flour. The amount of folate (folic acid) is higher in enriched white flour because it is added. (This chapter will explain why each of these nutrients is so important.)

	100% Whole-Grain Wheat Flour, 100 g	*Enriched, Bleached, All-Purpose White Flour, 100 g*
Calories, kcal	339.0	364.0
Dietary fiber, g	12.2	2.7
Calcium, mg	34.0	15.0
Magnesium, mg	138.0	22.0
Potassium, mg	405.0	107.0
Folate, DFE, mcg	44.0	291.0
Thiamin, mg	0.5	0.8
Riboflavin, mg	0.2	0.5
Niacin, mg	6.4	5.9
Iron, mg	3.9	4.6

Source: Agricultural Research Service Nutrient Database for Standard Reference, Release 17.[18]

How to Read a Label for Grain Content

The whole-grain health claim requires that the product be low-fat and that more than half its content be whole grain. Whole-grain product labels list whole grain as the first ingredient and the word whole *or* whole-grain *before the grain ingredient's name. They might also say* brown rice, bulgur, pearl barley, graham flour, quinoa, oatmeal, whole-grain corn, whole oats, whole rye, whole wheat, *or* wild rice. *Look for words that are listed in the "Whole Grain Foods" box on pages 47–48. The Percent Daily Value (% DV) for fiber is an additional clue to the amount of whole grain in the product. (See the discussion of Percent Daily Value in Chapter 7.) Choose products with a higher % DV for fiber. Products that have bran or grains added to them may have a very high fiber content but may lack the valuable nutrients from the germ. So look for the word* whole-grain *and buy products that list that ingredient first.*

Why Is the Grain Group Important?

Whole grains are an important source of fiber and nutrients. They raise our endurance level and help prevent

▲ Obesity, by supplying better nutrition and curbing the appetite

▲ Diabetes, by staying in the stomach longer, forestalling the increase in blood sugar

▲ Fatigue, malnutrition, and nervous system disorders, by supplying nutrients

▲ Cholesterol-related cardiovascular diseases

▲ Intestinal disorders, by improving elimination

Fiber Matters

Fiber is the bran on the outside of grain, the mostly indigestible cellulose. Although fiber provides little energy or caloric value, it serves other key roles. There are two kinds of dietary fiber: soluble and insoluble. Both are important for good health. Whereas other major grains like wheat, corn, and rice have predominantly insoluble fiber, oats, barley, and rye are good sources of soluble fiber.

Insoluble fiber passes through the body without dissolving. It optimizes intestinal function and the elimination of waste materials through the colon. Fiber is one of the best defenses against constipation, gastrointestinal disorders, diverticulosis, colon cancer, and appendicitis.

Soluble fiber (also called *beta-glucan*) dissolves in water. It forms a gel during digestion, prompting the liver to pull cholesterol out of the bloodstream. Hence, the body's overall cholesterol level diminishes. The effects of diets rich in soluble fiber appear most dramatic in those whose baseline blood cholesterol level is high.

Minerals

Iron transports oxygen in the blood. Grains help prevent iron-deficiency anemia, to which women of childbearing age are particularly susceptible. *Magnesium* builds bones and helps release energy from muscles. The germ of whole grains is loaded with *potassium,* which, with sodium, regulates the body's water base and acid base. It is vital for growth and muscle building. *Selenium,* an antioxidant, reinforces the immune system.

B Vitamins

The germ and bran of cereal grains are our best sources of *B vitamins: niacin, riboflavin, thiamin,* and *folate (folic acid).* In nature and in unrefined grains, these B vitamins occur together. Like spark plugs, they help the body unleash energy from the foods we eat by catalyzing many biochemical reactions. They optimize the function of the nervous system, counteracting stress, irritability, and fatigue. Hair, skin, and eyes also benefit from the B vitamins, as does liver function. Certain fats in our diet help optimize the B vitamins' utility.

Folate (folic acid) helps break down protein for cell generation. Pregnancy increases the requirement for folate as the fetus develops. Many refined-grain products are now folate enriched. As a result, unless whole grains are fortified with folic acid, they may actually have less folate than enriched refined grains. Look for folate-fortified whole-grain breakfast cereals.

Other Important Nutrients from Whole Grains

Lignans and *phytoestrogens* are estrogen-like substances found in some plants and plant products.

Phenolic compounds, or *polyphenols,* as they are also known, are powerful antioxidants—particularly the *flavonoids.* (See discussion of antioxidants on page 65.) In addition to fortifying the immune system, they help prevent heart disease and hypertension, and they strengthen the vascular system. Polyphenols also have an antibiotic and antiviral effect.

Another important substance found in whole grains is *phytic acid,* also called *inositol hexaphosphate.* All these nutrients contribute to staving off cancer.

Eating Lower
on the Food Chain

When people eat, they eat whatever those species that make up their food have been eating, as well as whatever chemicals they have absorbed from their environment. The animals at the top of the food chain, therefore, eat the highest concentrations of contaminants. Meat-eating humans are at the top. Pesticides and herbicides in livestock fodder end up in meat. Mercury from the ocean ends up in fish. One of the greatest advantages of eating more whole grains is that the grains, at the bottom of the food chain, have fewer contaminants. Substituting grains, vegetables, and produce for animal products reduces the level of pesticides consumed.

How Much Grain Should You Eat Daily?

Most of us eat plenty of grains, but too few of them are whole grains. *Remember, at least half of all the grains you eat should be whole.* The first step is figuring out how much grain you should be eating. The second step is determining the best way to make sure half of it is whole grain.

Look at the following chart. These are the minimum daily recommendations for people who get *less* than thirty minutes of moderate physical activity a day. More-active people will require more. My Pyramid recommends at least thirty minutes of moderate exercise daily, as part of a healthy regime.

		Daily Recommendation	Daily Minimum Amount of Whole Grains
Children	2–3 years old	3 oz. eq.	1½ oz. eq.
	4–8 years old	4–5 oz. eq.	2–2½ oz. eq.
Girls	9–13 years old	5 oz. eq.	3 oz. eq.
	14–18 years old	6 oz. eq.	3 oz. eq.
Boys	9–13 years old	6 oz. eq.	3 oz. eq.
	14–18 years old	7 oz. eq.	3½ oz. eq.
Women	19–30 years old	6 oz. eq.	3 oz. eq.
	31–50 years old	6 oz. eq.	3 oz. eq.
	51+ years old	5 oz. eq.	3 oz. eq.
Men	19–30 years old	8 oz. eq.	4 oz. eq.
	31–50 years old	7 oz. eq.	3½ oz. eq.
	51+ years old	6 oz. eq.	3 oz. eq.

What Is an Ounce Equivalent?

Ounce equivalent *is My Pyramid's way of quantifying its grain serving size recommendations. The word* serving *was used in the previous Food Pyramid. It was a tricky term because no one seemed to know exactly how much constituted a serving. My Pyramid tries to be more precise with its ounce equivalent.*

The term ounce equivalent *is based on the dry measurement of the grain portion of any given food. Instead of saying "ounce," it says "ounce equivalent." This is difficult to calculate without knowing how much grain is in the food you are eating. You must also know how much the grain weighs. (See the following chart for help.) To guess how many ounce equivalents a food item that is not on the list might be, you always need to think in terms of the weight of the grain that went into it. You really need the chart.*

How Much Grain Do Foods Contain?

In general, 1 slice of bread, 1 cup of ready-to-eat cereal, or ½ cup of cooked rice, cooked pasta, or cooked cereal is a 1 ounce equivalent from the Grains Group. This means that each contains 1 ounce of grain.

The following chart lists specific amounts that count as 1 ounce equivalent of grains toward your daily recommended intake. In some cases the number of ounce equivalents for common portions is also shown.

		Amount That Counts as 1 Ounce Equivalent of Grains	*Common Portions and Ounce Equivalents*
Bagels	WG*: whole wheat RG*: plain, egg	½ mini bagel	1 large bagel = 4 oz. eq.
Biscuits	(baking powder/ buttermilk—RG*)	1 small (2″ diameter)	1 large (3″ diameter) = 2 oz. eq.
Breads	WG*: 100% whole wheat RG*: white, wheat, French, sourdough	1 regular slice, 1 small slice French, 4 snack-size slices rye bread	2 regular slices = 2 oz. eq.
Bulgur	cracked wheat (WG*)	½ cup cooked	
Corn bread	(RG*)	1 small piece (2½″ × 1¼″ × 1¼″)	1 medium piece (2½″ × 2½″ × 1¼″) = 2 oz. eq.
Crackers	WG*: 100% whole wheat, rye	5 whole wheat crackers, 2 rye	

	RG*: saltines, snack crackers	crispbreads 7 square or round crackers	
English muffins	WG*: whole wheat RG*: plain, raisin	½ muffin	1 muffin = 2 oz. eq.
Muffins	WG*: whole wheat RG*: bran, corn, plain	1 small (2½" diameter)	1 large (3½" diameter) = 3 oz. eq.
Oatmeal	(WG)	½ cup cooked, 1 packet instant, 1 oz. dry (regular or quick)	
Pancakes	WG*: whole wheat, buckwheat RG*: buttermilk, plain	1 pancake (4 ½" diameter), 2 small pancakes (3" diameter)	3 pancakes (4 ½" diameter) = 3 oz. eq.
Popcorn	(WG*)	3 cups, popped bag, popped = 4 oz. eq.	1 microwave
Ready-to-eat breakfast cereal	WG*: toasted oat, whole wheat flakes RG*: cornflakes, puffed rice	1 cup flakes or rounds, 1¼ cup puffed	
Rice	WG*: brown, wild RG*: enriched, white, polished	½ cup cooked, 1 oz. dry	1 cup cooked = 2 oz. eq.
Pasta— spaghetti, macaroni, noodles	WG*: whole wheat RG*: enriched, durum	½ cup cooked, 1 oz. dry	1 cup cooked = 2 oz. eq.
Tortillas	WG*: whole wheat, whole-grain corn RG*: flour, corn	1 small flour tortilla (6" diameter) 1 corn tortilla (6" diameter)	1 large tortilla (12" diameter) = 4 oz. eq.

*WG = whole grains, RG = refined grains. This is shown when products are available both in whole-grain and refined-grain forms.

TIPS: Working Those Great Whole Grains into Your Diet

For most of us, the conversion from refined to whole grains takes some work. Do not just add whole grains to your diet of pasta and sweet rolls. *Substitute* whole-grain products for refined products. Out with the white bread; in with the whole-wheat bread. Exit white rice and white pasta; enter brown rice and whole-wheat pasta. Buy whole-grain cereal instead of refined cereal, or just eat oatmeal. Snack on whole-grain tortilla chips or popcorn with little or no butter or salt. Freeze leftover cooked brown rice, bulgur, or barley. Heat and serve later as a quick side dish or sprinkle in salads and soups.

This may seem, literally, a lot to chew on at first. However, a whole-grain cereal for breakfast and a whole-grain sandwich at lunch with two slices of bread meets the minimum adult recommendation. You might try using whole grains in combination with refined grains. Mix wild rice or brown rice with white rice. Use some whole-wheat, rye, or oat flour added to enriched white flour, in pancakes, breads, piecrust, and muffins. Since whole-grain flours are heavier, it will affect the rising and cooking time and may require more leavening. Make cookies that include whole-grain flours for snacks. Experiment. The grain portion need not be the entire meal. Here are some suggestions to get you started:

▲ Stuff baked green peppers or tomatoes with brown rice or tabouli (bulgur).

▲ Serve whole-wheat macaroni and cheese.

▲ Add barley to vegetable soup or stews.

▲ Use bulgur wheat in casseroles or stir-fries.

▲ Make whole-grain pilaf with a mixture of barley, wild rice, brown rice, broth, and spices. For a special touch, stir in toasted nuts or chopped dried fruit.

▲ Use whole-grain bread or cracker crumbs in meat loaf.

▲ Bread chicken, fish, veal cutlets, or eggplant parmesan in rolled oats or a crushed, unsweetened whole grain cereal and bake.

▲ Use unsweetened, whole-grain ready-to-eat cereal as croutons in salad or in place of crackers with soup.

Whole Grains for Children

Children are usually fussier eaters than adults, but they also have demanding nutritional requirements. Therefore, set a good example by eating and serving whole grains with meals and snacks. To increase their enthusiasm, let children select and help prepare whole-grain dishes. Teach them to identify whether whole grains are at the top of the ingredient list on cereal and snack food packages.

The Vegetable Group

My Pyramid Directive: **Generally, adults should consume 2.5 or more cups of vegetables per day. This allotment varies slightly according to gender, age, and activity level. Toddlers require only 1 cup of vegetables, a requirement that grows as they mature.**

What Is the Vegetable Group?

On the My Pyramid graphic, the green segment to the right of the Grain Group represents the Vegetable Group, which is packed with vitamins and minerals. Any vegetable or 100 percent vegetable juice counts as a member of the Vegetable Group. Vegetables may be raw or cooked and fresh, frozen, canned, or dried/dehydrated. Whole, cut up, or mashed, they can be eaten as main courses; in salads, soups, and side dishes; or as snacks.

My Pyramid organizes vegetables into five categories based on their nutrient content. Moving between categories and mixing your meals from among these different veggies ensures that you will be getting better nutritional value from the food you eat. Varying their preparation and using seasonings turns them into tasty additions that can help you lower your fat intake. Here are the categories. Each list starts with the most nutrient-packed vegetable.

Dark Green Vegetables

These carotenoid-rich sources of vitamin A and vitamin C are probably the healthiest foods on earth. They are also packed with calcium, magnesium, and potassium, with traces of copper, manganese, and zinc. With the exception of folate (folic acid), they are low in B vitamins. This abundance of nutrients is due largely to chlorophyll. Chlorophyll delivers essential fuel to plants as blood does in humans. It is especially concentrated in green, leafy vegetables that thrive in the sunshine. Obviously, chlorophyll is good for humans, too.

Bok choy

Broccoli

Collard greens

Dark green leafy lettuce

Kale

Mesclun

Mustard greens

Romaine lettuce

Spinach

Turnip greens

Watercress

Beet greens

Chard

Dandelion greens

Orange Vegetables

These vegetables derive their volumes of vitamin A from beta-carotene. They also contain vitamin C, potassium, calcium, iron, and magnesium. High in carbohydrates and fiber, they can be more filling than other vegetables.

Acorn squash

Butternut squash

Carrots

Hubbard squash

Pumpkin

Sweet potatoes

Beans and Peas

This category includes dry beans and canned beans. Mainly a mixture of protein and starch, these legumes are low in fat and calories—a high-quality complex carbohydrate. They have some B vitamins and iron, calcium, potassium, and phosphorus.

Black beans

Black-eyed peas

Garbanzo beans (chickpeas)

Adzuki beans (also known as azuki and aduki beans)

Great northern beans

Mung beans

Kidney beans

Lentils

Lima beans (mature)

Navy beans

Pinto beans

Soybeans

Split peas

Tofu (bean curd made from soybeans)

White beans

Starchy Vegetables

These hardy vegetables are high in carbohydrates but also contain reasonable amounts of vitamin C and the B vitamins (especially folate), potassium, magnesium, manganese, iron, and zinc. Corn, green peas, and lima beans have good quantities of vitamin A. Technically, corn is a grain, but My Pyramid classifies it in the Vegetable Group.

Corn

Green peas

Lima beans (green)

Potatoes

Other Vegetables

This catchall category has more of what's good for us. It is composed of the cruciferous vegetables (edible plant flowers—cauliflower, Brussels sprouts), stem vegetables (asparagus, celery, leeks, rhubarb), roots (beets, parsnips, rutabagas), and miscellaneous vegetables and fruits. All are good sources of nutrients and high in fiber.

Artichokes

Asparagus

Bean sprouts

Beets

Brussels sprouts

Cabbage

Cauliflower

Celery

Cucumbers

Eggplant

Green beans

Green and red peppers

Iceberg (head) lettuce

Leeks

Mushrooms

Okra

Onions

Parsnips

Rutabagas

Tomatoes

Tomato juice

Vegetable juice

Turnips

Wax beans

Zucchini

Why Is the Vegetable Group Important?

Proof that Americans are not eating their fresh vegetables is apparent from the disease and mortality statistics cited in Chapter 1. Our sedentary, stress-filled lifestyles and our increasingly

Vegetables from the Sea

My Pyramid does not make reference to ocean vegetables, even though they are extremely high in iodine, iron, calcium, and potassium. This oversight may be due to the fact that they are more popular in other cultures than in the United States. Common seaweed products are kelp, nori, dulse, agar-agar, arame, hijiki, kombu, and wakame. Algin is a fiber molecule in most seaweeds that attracts heavy metals in our bodies and carries them out through elimination.[19]

contaminated environment combine to sabotage good health. Occasionally plunging corn chips into the bean dip is not enough. Americans must buckle down and eat more vegetables! Vegetables are our best defense against chronic diseases.

Since vegetables are low in calories and high in fiber, they are a great diet food. Furthermore, they contain no cholesterol. Including abundant vegetables in a balanced diet may reduce the risk of

▲ Stroke, coronary heart disease, and other cardiovascular diseases

▲ Type 2 diabetes

▲ Certain cancers, such as mouth, stomach, and colorectal cancer

▲ Developing kidney stones

▲ Bone disease

▲ High blood pressure

Antioxidants

The antioxidant story begins with free radicals, which are produced by stress and exposure to pollutants. These unstable molecules cause oxidization in living systems, damaging cells and disturbing their ability to function normally. The result of the oxidation is depleted immunity, leaving the body vulnerable to disease. Antioxidants are among the large group of phytochemicals (chemicals found naturally in plants) that have a positive effect on health. They protect the cells against the harmful influence of free radicals. Vitamins A, C, and E and other plant chemicals have an antioxidant effect.

Vitamins

Nutrient-rich vegetables contain antioxidants that can put a stop to destruction caused by free radicals. *Antioxidants*—in the form of *vitamins A, C,* and *E*—neutralize free radicals by donating electrons to the atoms in the cells and returning the cells to stability. But do not think you can merely substitute doses of these vitamins for your greens. Other chemicals and substances found in *natural* sources of antioxidants seem to enable the beneficial effects. The combined substances provide greater protection than that of any single nutrient or individual antioxidant supplement. Moreover, no one yet knows the long-term effect of large doses of these nutrients. A balanced diet with lots of vegetables is still our best fortifier. The more nutrients we eat, the better stoked our bodies are to do their job in a world of invisible environmental peril.

Beta-carotene is the best known of the *carotenoids,* the red, orange, and yellow pigments that give color to many vegetables (and fruits). The body converts beta-carotene into *vitamin A,* now recognized as vital to the growth and development of the human body. Vitamin A is also a potent immune-system booster and a powerful antioxidant.

Vitamin C is the most abundant water-soluble antioxidant in the body. Vitamin C helps heal cuts and wounds and keeps teeth and gums healthy. In addition, it aids iron absorption and returns vitamin E to its active form. Unfortunately, it passes through the body very quickly, and as an unstable vitamin (more about this in Chapter 8), it dissipates from food very quickly, often before it is consumed. This is one reason why it is prudent to eat produce so many times a day.

Vitamin E is the most abundant fat-soluble antioxidant. Although it can come from vegetables, most of it ends up in vegetable oils (see the discussion of the Oils Group later in this chapter). Uncooked green peas, soybeans, spinach, asparagus, kale, cucumber, tomato, and celery have some vitamin E.

Although vegetables, with the exception of legumes, are low in B vitamins, they are a good source of *folate* (*folic acid*). Folate plays a part in the formation of red blood cells and is particularly important to pregnant women. It reduces the risk of neural tube defects, spina bifida, and brain defects during fetal development.[20]

Minerals

Vegetables are very high in minerals; however, the amount varies depending on the condition of the soil in which they are grown and on their storage and preparation. This makes it all the more important to purchase high-quality fresh produce. Remember Popeye and his secret weapon—spinach? Green leafy vegetables are packed with *iron, magnesium, potassium,* and other *minerals.* Cruciferous vegetables and legumes are great sources of calcium, which works in defense of strong bones.

Fiber

The indigestible fibrous parts of vegetables are an important aspect of our dietary fiber (see "Fiber Matters" in the Grains Group section earlier in this chapter). They help lower blood cholesterol levels and may thus lower the risk of heart disease. Fiber reduces constipation and optimizes elimination.

How Many Vegetables Should You Eat Daily?

Minimum recommended total daily amounts for people who get *less* than thirty minutes per day of moderate physical activity are shown in the following table. More-active people will require greater amounts. My Pyramid recommends at least thirty minutes of moderate exercise daily, as part of a healthy regime.

Daily Recommendation

Children	2–3 years old	1 cup
	4–8 years old	1½ cups
Girls	9–13 years old	2 cups
	14–18 years old	2½ cups
Boys	9–13 years old	2½ cups
	14–18 years old	3 cups
Women	19–30 years old	2½ cups
	31–50 years old	2½ cups
	51+ years old	2 cups
Men	19–30 years old	3 cups
	31–50 years old	3 cups
	51+ years old	2½ cups

Recommendations follow for how much to eat from each vegetable subgroup on a weekly basis. It is not necessary to eat vegetables from each subgroup daily. However, over the course of a week, try to consume the amounts listed from each subgroup as a way to reach your daily intake recommendation.

	Dark Green Vegetables	Orange Vegetables	Dry Beans and Peas	Starchy Vegetables	Other Vegetables
			Amount Per Week		
Children					
2–3 years old	1 cup	½ cup	½ cup	1½ cups	4 cups
4–8 years old	1½ cups	1 cup	1 cup	2½ cups	4½ cups
Girls					
9–13 years old	2 cups	1½ cups	2½ cups	2½ cups	5½ cups
14–18 years old	3 cups	2 cups	3 cups	3 cups	6½ cups
Boys					
9–13 years old	3 cups	2 cups	3 cups	3 cups	6½ cups
14–18 years old	3 cups	2 cups	3 cups	6 cups	7 cups
Women					
19–30 years old	3 cups	2 cups	3 cups	3 cups	6½ cups
31–50 years old	3 cups	2 cups	3 cups	3 cups	6½ cups
51+ years old	2 cups	1½ cups	2½ cups	2½ cups	5½ cups
Men					
19–30 years old	3 cups	2 cups	3 cups	6 cups	7 cups
31–50 years old	3 cups	2 cups	3 cups	6 cups	7 cups
51+ years old	3 cups	2 cups	3 cups	3 cups	6½ cups

How Much Is a Cup?

In My Pyramid vegetable recommendations, a cup is mostly a cup, about the size of a fist. The exception is raw leafy greens; 2 cups of raw leafy greens are equivalent to 1 cup, as you will see in the following chart.

	Amount That Counts as 1 Cup of Vegetables	*Amount That Counts as ½ Cup of Vegetables*
Dark green vegetables		
Broccoli	1 cup chopped or florets 3 spears 5″ long Raw or cooked	

Greens (collards, mustard greens, turnip greens, kale)	1 cup, cooked	
Spinach	1 cup, cooked 2 cups raw is equivalent to 1 cup of vegetables	1 cup raw is equivalent to ½ cup of vegetables
Raw leafy greens (spinach, romaine, watercress, dark green leafy lettuce, endive, escarole)	2 cups raw is equivalent to 1 cup of vegetables	1 cup raw is equivalent to ½ cup of vegetables

Orange vegetables

Carrots	1 cup, strips, slices, or chopped, raw or cooked 2 medium 1 cup baby carrots (about 12)	1 medium carrot About 6 baby carrots
Pumpkin	1 cup mashed, cooked	
Sweet potato	1 large baked (2¼″ or more diameter) 1 cup sliced or mashed, cooked	
Winter squash (acorn, butternut, hubbard)	1 cup cubed, cooked	½ acorn squash, baked = ¾ cup

Dry beans and peas

Dry beans and peas (black, garbanzo, kidney, pinto, or soybeans) or black-eyed peas or split peas	1 cup whole or mashed, cooked	
Tofu	1 cup ½″ cubes (about 8 oz.)	1 piece 2½″ × 2¾″ × 1″ (about 4 oz.)

Starchy vegetables

Corn, yellow or white	1 cup 1 large ear (8″–9″ long)	1 small ear (about 6″ long)

	Amount That Counts as 1 Cup of Vegetables	*Amount That Counts as ½ Cup of Vegetables*
Green peas	1 cup	
White potatoes	1 cup diced, mashed 1 medium boiled or baked potato (2½"–3" diameter) French-fried: 20 medium to long strips (2½"–4" long) (Contains discretionary calories.)	

Other vegetables

	Amount That Counts as 1 Cup of Vegetables	*Amount That Counts as ½ Cup of Vegetables*
Bean sprouts	1 cup, cooked	
Cabbage, green	1 cup, chopped or shredded, raw or cooked	
Cauliflower	1 cup pieces or florets, raw or cooked	
Celery	1 cup, diced or sliced, raw or cooked 2 large stalks (11"–12" long)	1 large stalk (11"–12" long)
Cucumbers	1 cup raw, sliced or chopped	
Green or wax beans	1 cup cooked	
Green or red peppers	1 cup chopped, raw or cooked 1 large pepper (3" diameter, 3¾" long)	1 small pepper
Lettuce, iceberg or head	2 cups raw, shredded or chopped is equivalent to 1 cup of vegetables	1 cup raw, shredded or chopped is equivalent to ½ cup of vegetables
Mushrooms	1 cup, raw or cooked	
Onions	1 cup chopped, raw or cooked	
Tomatoes	1 large raw whole (3")	1 small, raw, whole (2¼")

	1 cup chopped or sliced, raw, canned, or cooked	1 medium, canned
Tomato or mixed vegetable juice	1 cup	½ cup
Summer squash or zucchini	1 cup cooked, sliced or diced	

Tips: Working Those Revitalizing Vegetables into Your Diet

Buying fresh vegetables in season—from farmers markets and other vendors of local produce—means you will be getting more flavor and more nutrient value . . . and likely at a better price. The downside is that fresh vegetables take longer to prepare, which is a big reason that busy people are less likely to get their full 2.5 cups daily. The following tips may help get the fresh vegetables to your mouth more easily. Frozen vegetables are second best.

Safety Tips

To remove dirt and surface microorganisms, wash vegetables before preparing and eating. Use clean, running water. Rub vegetables briskly with your hands or a vegetable brush. Dry after washing. Keep vegetables separate from raw meat, poultry, and seafood while shopping, preparing, and storing. Do not use the same cutting board for vegetables that you use for raw meat.

To save time:

▲ On a weekend, prepare a big pot of homemade vegetable soup that you and your family can enjoy all week.

▲ In warmer months, keep a pitcher of gazpacho (spicy, cold chopped vegetable soup) or vichyssoise (cold leek and potato soup) in the refrigerator.

▲ Lightly steam, stir-fry, or sauté a large quantity of vegetables once or twice a week that you can reheat or eat cold for several days.

▲ Purchase prewashed bags of salad greens and other vegetables.

▲ Carrots, celery, cherry tomatoes, cauliflower, red and green peppers, and broccoli pieces make easy, healthful snacks. Keep them in a transparent container to motivate you to eat them. Serve them with bean dip, spinach dip, hummus (chickpea dip), or salsa to increase your vegetable intake.

▲ Steam a big batch of leafy greens right when you get home from the grocery store, then freeze it until you can heat up a portion with sautéed garlic and other seasonings.

▲ Hydrate flaked, dried legumes (black beans, split peas, etc.) with broth and seasonings to make quick soups and side dishes.

To incorporate more vegetables into your diet:

▲ Keep parsley, cilantro, and other favorite herbs on hand. Chop and use as edible garnishes.

▲ Use grated carrots and zucchini in meat loaf, casseroles, quick breads, and muffins.

▲ Eat a green salad every night after the main course and before dessert, as the French do.

▲ Use puréed cooked vegetables to thicken stews, soups, gravies, and sauces.

▲ Include vegetables in pasta sauce and on pizzas.

▲ Grill vegetables (eggplant, tomatoes, mushrooms, peppers, onions) when you grill meat or tofu.

Go Easy on the Fat

Try not to undo all the good you are doing in eating no-fat vegetables by cooking them in quantities of fat or adding rich sauces. (The Fat Group section, later in this chapter, makes suggestions for low-fat sauces, toppings, dips, and spreads.)

Making Vegetables Appealing to Children

▲ Set a good example by eating and serving vegetables with meals and as snacks.

▲ Let children decide which vegetables to include in salads.

▲ Ask children to help pick out vegetables at the market. They might also enjoy washing, peeling, and cutting them.

▲ Invite children to choose one new vegetable when you shop together.

▲ If children do not like their vegetables mixed with each other or with other foods, serve vegetables as side dishes.

The Fruit Group

My Pyramid Directive: Generally, adults should consume 2 or more cups of fruit per day. This allotment varies slightly according to your gender, age, and activity level. Toddlers require only 1 cup of fruit, a requirement that grows as they mature.

What Is the Fruit Group?

On the My Pyramid graphic, the red segment to the right of the Vegetable Group represents the Fruit Group. Any fruit or 100 percent fruit juice counts as a member of the Fruit Group. Fruits may be raw or cooked, fresh, frozen, canned, or dried/dehydrated. Whole, cut-up, or mashed, they can be eaten with cereals, salads, side dishes, desserts, or snacks.

Fruits contain plentiful vitamins, minerals, and fiber, but they are also high in sugar content. Low in fat as well as high in fiber and sugar, fruits make a good substitute for sugary desserts and snacks. Fruit juices are, of course, preferable to soda.

Miscellaneous Fruit

Apples

Apricots

Avocados

Bananas

Figs

Grapes

Kiwifruit

Mangoes

Nectarines

Oranges

Papaya

Peaches

Pears

Persimmon

Pineapple

Plums

Pomegranate

Berries

Blueberries

Boysenberries

Cherries

Cranberries

Currants

Gooseberries

Lingonberries

Raspberries

Strawberries

Citrus

Grapefruit

Lemons

Limes

Oranges

Tangerines

Melons

Cantaloupe

Casaba

Crenshaw

Honeydew

Watermelon

Mixed Fruit

Fruit cocktail (unsweetened)

Dried Fruit

Apples

Apricots

Blueberries

Cherries

Cranberries

Dates

Figs

Peaches

Pears

Prunes

Raisins

Strawberries

100 Percent Fruit Juice

Any fruit can be juiced, and fruit juices of enormous variety are available year-round. The more recently they were juiced, the more nutritious they are. Beware of "juice cocktails," which contain added sugar.

The Juice Story

Fruit juice is nutritious but does not impart the dietary fiber benefits, as do whole and pared fruit. Purchase 100 percent fruit juice, rather than juice made from concentrate. To get the benefit of fiber plus the added nutrients of fresh fruit, make sure to eat whole fruit in addition to fruit juice.

Why Is the Fruit Group Important?

If you are old enough to remember the adage "an apple a day keeps the doctor away," you already know that eating fruit is good for you. Yet today too many people come no closer to a fruit than having a fruit-flavored soda or maybe a glass of OJ, even though today's food markets offer more diversity and quantities of fruit than ever before. Fruit juice is a perfectly viable segment of the Fruit Group, but it is whole fresh fruit that delivers the greatest benefit—to our health, our looks, and our mental outlook.

Fruits are low in fat and have no cholesterol. Including abundant fruits in a balanced diet may reduce the risk of

▲ Stroke, coronary heart disease, and other cardiovascular diseases

▲ Type 2 diabetes

▲ Certain cancers, such as mouth, stomach, and colorectal cancer

▲ Developing kidney stones

▲ Bone disease

▲ High blood pressure

▲ Unwanted weight gain

Detoxification is a normal body process of eliminating or neutralizing toxins through the colon, liver, kidneys, lungs, lymph glands, and skin. Because fruits are high in fiber and water content, and they increase the speed at which food moves through the intestine, they are easy to digest. Passing through the body quickly, they have a relatively low allergenic potential.

Vitamins

Fruits deliver the same antioxidant vitamins as vegetables, containing vitamins A, C, and in the seeds, vitamin E. *Vitamin A,* in the form of beta-carotene, gives many fruits their red, orange, and yellow color. (See the box "Antioxidants" in the Vegetable Group section earlier in this chapter)

Vitamin C is particularly abundant in citrus fruits—oranges, lemons, grapefruit, tangerines, and limes. We have long known that vitamin C has an immune-enhancing role; now we know these are antioxidants at work. In addition to its antioxidant function, vitamin C contributes to the growth and repair of body tissues. It also keeps teeth and gums healthy. Vitamin C courses through the body very quickly and is used up even more rapidly under stressful conditions or during exposure to smoking, alcohol, or poor environmental conditions—proof-positive that it is doing its job. Nevertheless, it is imperative to keep up your supply of vitamin C by eating fruits (and vegetables) as often as possible.

Like vegetables, fruits are low in B vitamins, but they are still a good source of *folate* (*folic acid*). Folate plays a part in the formation of red blood cells and is particularly important to pregnant women. It reduces the risk of neural tube defects, spina bifida, and brain damage during fetal development.[21]

Fiber

The indigestible fibrous parts of fruits are an important aspect of our *dietary fiber.* (See "Fiber Matters" in the Grains Group section earlier in this chapter.) Fiber helps reduce blood cholesterol levels and may thus lower the risk of heart disease. Fiber reduces constipation and optimizes elimination. Since fruits are low in calories and high in fiber, they are a great diet food.

Minerals

Fruits are an important source of several minerals, including *calcium, magnesium, copper,* and *manganese,* a little *iron,* and other *trace minerals,* though quantities vary depending on the soil in which they are grown. They also contain *potassium,* which is vital for growth and muscle building. Chemically, potassium regulates the body's water base and acid base. Bananas, prunes, dried peaches and apricots, cantaloupe, honeydew melon, and orange juice are all loaded with potassium.

How Many Fruits Should You Eat Daily?

Minimum recommended total daily amounts for people who get *less* than thirty minutes per day of moderate physical activity are shown in the following chart. More-active people will require greater amounts. My Pyramid recommends at least thirty minutes of moderate exercise daily, as part of a healthy regime.

		Daily Recommendation
Children	2–3 years old	1 cup
	4–8 years old	1 to 1½ cups
Girls	9–13 years old	1½ cups
	14–18 years old	1½ cups
Boys	9–13 years old	1½ cups
	14–18 years old	2 cups
Women	19–30 years old	2 cups
	31–50 years old	1½ cups
	51+ years old	1½ cups
Men	19–30 years old	2 cups
	31–50 years old	2 cups
	51+ years old	2 cups

How Much Is a Cup?

In My Pyramid fruit recommendations, a cup is mostly a cup, about the size of a fist. The exception is dried fruit, in which ½ cup is considered to be 1 cup from the Fruit Group. The following specific amounts count as 1 cup of fruit (in some cases equivalents for ½ cup are also shown) toward your Daily Recommended Intake.

	Amount That Counts as 1 Cup of Fruit	*Amount That Counts as ½ Cup of Fruit*
Apple	½ large (3.25″ diameter) 1 small (2.5″ diameter) 1 cup sliced or chopped, raw or cooked	½ cup sliced or chopped, raw or cooked
Applesauce	1 cup	1 snack container (4 oz.)
Banana	1 cup sliced 1 large (8″–9″ long)	1 small (less than 6″ long)
Cantaloupe	1 cup diced or melon balls	1 medium wedge (⅛ of a medium melon)
Grapes	1 cup whole or cut up 32 seedless grapes	16 seedless grapes
Grapefruit	1 medium (4″ diameter) 1 cup sections	½ medium (4″ diameter)
Mixed fruit (fruit cocktail)	1 cup diced or sliced, raw or canned, drained	1 snack container (4 oz.) drained = ⅜ cup
Orange	1 large (3¹⁄₁₆″ diameter) 1 cup sections	1 small (2⅜″ diameter)
Orange, mandarin	1 cup canned, drained	
Peach	1 large (2¾″ diameter) 1 cup sliced or diced, raw, cooked, or canned, drained 2 halves, canned	1 small (2″ diameter) 1 snack container (4 oz.) drained = ⅜ cup
Pear	1 medium pear (2.5 per lb.) 1 cup sliced or diced, raw, cooked, or canned, drained	1 snack container (4 oz.) drained = ⅜ cup
Pineapple	1 cup chunks, sliced or crushed, raw, cooked or canned, drained	1 snack container (4 oz.) drained = ⅜ cup
Plum	1 cup sliced raw or cooked 3 medium or 2 large plums	1 large plum

Strawberries	About 8 large berries 1 cup whole, halved, or sliced, fresh or frozen	½ cup whole, halved, or sliced
Watermelon	1 small wedge (1″ thick) 1 cup diced or balls	6 melon balls
Dried fruit (raisins, prunes, apricots, etc.)	½ cup dried fruit is equivalent to 1 cup fruit, ½ cup raisins, ½ cup prunes, ½ cup dried apricots	¼ cup dried fruit is equivalent to ½ cup fruit, 1 small box raisins (1.5 oz.)
100% fruit juice (orange, apple, grape, grapefruit, etc.)	1 cup	½ cup

Tips: Working Those Revitalizing Fruits into Your Diet

Shopping Tips

Buying fresh fruits in season—preferably from farmers markets and other vendors of local produce—means you will be getting

Safety Tips

To remove dirt and surface microorganisms, wash fruits before preparing and eating. Use clean, running water. Rub fruits briskly with your hands or a vegetable brush. Dry after washing. Keep fruits separate from raw meat, poultry, and seafood while shopping, preparing, and storing. Do not use the same cutting board for fruits that you use for raw meat.

more flavor and more nutrient value . . . and likely at a better price.

Buy prepared fruits, either dried or frozen, without added sugar. Sulfur dioxide and other sulfites are effective preservatives used in dried and canned fruit; however, some people are allergic to them. The healthiest canned fruits are packaged in water or fruit juice rather than sugary syrup. Read labels.

Save time by buying prechopped fruit in bags.

Other Time-Saving Tips to Encourage More Fruit Eating

▲ Keep a bowl of whole fruit on the counter or table, as well as in the refrigerator, where you and your family will see and be motivated to eat it.

▲ After shopping, wash, pare, chop, and mix a variety of fruits. Refrigerate the fruit compote in a transparent container, to inspire you and your family to enjoy it all week. Unless it contains citrus fruits, squeeze some lemon juice or orange juice over it so the fruits do not discolor.

▲ Serve chopped fruits on top of cereal in the morning, together with a glass of fruit juice.

▲ Send your children to school with canned fruit juices or fresh bottled fruit juice, rather than sodas or other sweetened beverages. Take these to work with you, too.

▲ Pack whole fruits or container fruits in lunches.

▲ Make fruit smoothies for breakfast beverages or as snacks.

▲ Serve dried fruits as snacks instead of candy.

▲ Serve fruit on skewers using a variety of fruit.

▲ Frozen juice bars are a great hot-weather snack.

▲ Peanut butter and flavored yogurt are healthy toppings for breakfast, snacks, or desserts.

▲ Keep packages of dried fruit in your bag and at work for pick-me-ups.

▲ Include fruits in salads, and use fruit vinegar in the dressings.

▲ Incorporate fruits into bread, muffin, waffle, French toast, and pancake recipes.

▲ Add fruit to meat, poultry, and fish dishes.

▲ Use chopped fruit toppings on pancakes, waffles, French toast, and desserts.

▲ Use fruits as desserts, such as baked apples, poached pears, and fresh fruit pies.

▲ Serve a basket of fruit after dinner instead of dessert.

Fruit Ideas for Children

▲ Set a good example by eating and serving fruits with meals and as snacks.

▲ Let children decide which fruits to use as snacks and desserts.

▲ Ask children to help pick out fruits at the market. They might also enjoy washing, peeling, and cutting them.

▲ Invite children to choose one new fruit when you shop together.

The Milk Group

My Pyramid Directive: **Generally, adults should consume three or more portions (cup equivalents) of fat-free or low-fat milk products per day. This allotment varies slightly according to gender, age, and activity level. Toddlers require only two portions of milk products, a requirement that grows as they mature.**

What Is the Milk Group?

On the My Pyramid graphic, the large blue segment to the right of the Oils Group represents the Milk Group, containing the milk, yogurt, and cheese that come from cows. Its proportions are slightly larger than they were on the previous Food Pyramid. My Pyramid touts the calcium these foods offer and prioritizes low-fat offerings. It omits foods that have little calcium, such as cream cheese, cream, and butter. (Butter is in the Oils Group.)

Milk

Fat-free (skim)

Low-fat (1 percent)

Reduced-fat (2 percent)

Whole milk

Chocolate milk

Strawberry milk

Lactose-reduced milk

Lactose-free milk

Milk-Based Desserts

Puddings and custards made with milk

Ice milk

Frozen yogurt

Ice cream

Cheese

Cheddar

Mozzarella

Swiss

Parmesan and other hard cheeses

Ricotta

Cottage cheese and other soft cheeses

Yogurt

Fat-free

Low-fat

Reduced-fat

Whole-milk yogurt

Why Low-Fat Dairy Products?

As animal products, all dairy foods have saturated fats in them before they are processed. Saturated fats lead to more than unwanted calories. They raise levels of bad cholesterol—low-density lipoproteins, or LDLs. Higher levels of LDLs increase vulnerability to heart disease, hypertension, and stroke. Whole milk, many cheeses, and whole-milk yogurt are high in saturated fat. To help maintain healthy weight and blood cholesterol levels, keep these foods to a minimum.

Why Is the Milk Group Important?

Dairy products are not for everyone, yet they remain an important source of nutrients for many Americans, contributing to

the body's health and maintenance. Of course, babies and growing children often benefit from milk because it builds strong
bones and teeth. Now, as our population remains active and lives
longer, we have become aware that milk products can help reduce the risk of osteoporosis on the other end of life.

Vitamins

Vitamin D is essential because it helps regulate calcium metabolism and regulates our use of phosphorous. Vitamin D is a fat-
soluble substance, also known as the "sunshine vitamin"
because our bodies manufacture it when in contact with ultra-
violet light. When ingested, for instance with dairy products
(and some seafood), it is absorbed through the intestinal walls.

Vitamin A is also a potent immune-system booster and a
powerful antioxidant; however, it is most available in whole-
milk products.

Minerals

Calcium is the most abundant mineral in the human body, almost all of it in our bones. This explains why calcium-rich milk
is so important early in life, while bones are rapidly growing.
Calcium works in conjunction with magnesium to regulate
heart and muscle contraction. It optimizes nerve conduction
and the release of neurotransmitters. It is also necessary for cell
division. Bones provide calcium to the blood and other tissues.
An insufficient diet can deplete calcium reserves in the bones.
That the elderly tend to drink less milk and eat less well overall
increases their susceptibility to bone breakage and bone disease.

Potassium found in milk products—especially yogurt and
milk—helps maintain healthy blood pressure.

Bioavailability

Certain ingredients inhibit the absorption of some nutri-
ents. Others enhance it. Bioavailability is the amount of
nutrients that are actually absorbed. Because many of
milk's main nutrients—calcium, magnesium, phospho-
rous, and vitamin D—work together in good balance to
help their collective absorption from the digestive track,
they are said to increase bioavailability.

Lactose Intolerance

Most people of western European descent are able to safely
consume milk products all their lives, while most Africans,
Asians, southern Europeans, and the indigenous populations of
the Americas and the Pacific Islands cannot.[22] They are *lactose
intolerant*. Lactose intolerance occurs in people whose bodies
no longer have an enzyme called *lactase*. They lose the enzyme,
and with it the ability to digest milk, sometime during their
early childhood years. Lactase helps metabolize milk, and consuming milk without it may produce gas and diarrhea. It is
quite common for adults to be missing the enzyme, as the result of a genetic mutation many millennia ago.[23] People of
western European descent can digest milk because their ancestors consumed so many milk products that they retained the active enzyme into adulthood. Sometimes lactose intolerance
crops up in adulthood even in people of western European descent.

To accommodate ethnic diversity in the United States and
lactose-intolerant people who still enjoy dairy products, many
lactose-free and lower-lactose products are now available.

These include hard cheeses, ice cream, and yogurt. To accommodate vegans, some substitute soy milk, rice milk, and almond milk. Another recent solution is a pill that artificially provides the missing enzyme, allowing a person to tolerate milk products for a period of a few hours after taking it.

Bear in mind that one of the nutritional goals of including the Milk Group is to supply calcium. (This is not the only goal—milk products are a source of many nutrients supplying protein, phosphorus, etc.). Therefore, vegans and lactose-intolerant people can make up the different with calcium-rich foods, or calcium-fortified foods, such as soy beverages and orange juice. Milk products supply other nutrients, too, so those who do not consume them need to make up the difference in proteins, vitamins, and minerals with abundant selections from other food groups.

Nondairy Food Sources
of Calcium

Following are nondairy food sources of calcium, ranked by milligrams of calcium and calories per standard amount, but not by bioavailability *(the amount of calcium the body can absorb). The USDA has not published these figures but writes that "some plant foods have calcium that is well absorbed, but one has to eat a large quantity of vegetables to acquire as much calcium as is in a glass of milk." The USDA calls the amount we should be consuming daily the AI, which stands for* adequate intake. *For adults, the AI of calcium is 1,000 milligrams per day.*[24]

Food, Standard Amount	Calcium (mg)	Calories
Fortified ready-to-eat cereals (various), 1 oz.	236–1,043	88–106
Soy beverage, calcium fortified, 1 cup	368	98
Sardines, Atlantic, in oil, drained, 3 oz.	325	177
Tofu, firm, prepared with nigari,* ½ cup	253	88
Pink salmon, canned, with bone, 3 oz.	181	118
Collards, cooked from frozen, ½ cup	178	31
Molasses, blackstrap, 1 Tbsp.	172	47
Spinach, cooked from frozen, ½ cup	146	30
Soybeans, green, cooked, ½ cup	130	127
Turnip greens, cooked from frozen, ½ cup	124	24
Ocean perch, Atlantic, cooked, 3 oz.	116	103
Oatmeal, plain and flavored, instant, fortified, 1 packet prepared	99–110	97–157
Cowpeas, cooked, ½ cup	106	80
White beans, canned, ½ cup	96	153
Kale, cooked from frozen, ½ cup	90	20
Okra, cooked from frozen, ½ cup	88	26
Soybeans, mature, cooked, ½ cup	88	149
Blue crab, canned, 3 oz.	86	84
Beet greens, cooked from fresh, ½ cup	82	19
Bok choy, Chinese cabbage, cooked from fresh, ½ cup	79	10
Clams, canned, 3 oz.	78	126
Dandelion greens, cooked from fresh, ½ cup	74	17
Rainbow trout, farmed, cooked, 3 oz.	73	144

*Calcium sulfate and magnesium chloride.
Source: Dietary Guidelines for Americans, 2005, USDA.

How Many Milk Products Should You Eat Daily?

Minimum recommended total daily amounts for people who get *less* than thirty minutes per day of moderate physical activity are shown in the following chart. More-active people will require greater amounts. My Pyramid recommends at least thirty minutes of moderate exercise daily, as part of a healthy regime.

Daily Recommendation

Children	2–3 years old	2 cups
	4–8 years old	2 cups
Girls	9–13 years old	3 cups
	14–18 years old	3 cups
Boys	9–13 years old	3 cups
	14–18 years old	3 cups
Women	19–30 years old	3 cups
	31–50 years old	3 cups
	51+ years old	3 cups
Men	19–30 years old	3 cups
	31–50 years old	3 cups
	51+ years old	3 cups

How Much Is a Cup Equivalent?

Cup equivalent *is My Pyramid's way of quantifying its milk serving size recommendations. The word* serving *was used in the previous Food Pyramid. It was a tricky term because no one seemed to know exactly how much constituted a serving. My Pyramid tries to be more precise with its cup equivalent.*

The term cup equivalent *is based on measurement of the liquid milk portion of any given dairy food. Instead of saying* cup, *it says* cup equivalent. *This is difficult to calculate without knowing how much liquid milk went into the food you are eating. See the following chart for help.*

The following chart lists specific amounts that count as 1 cup in the Milk Group toward your Daily Recommended Intake.

	Amount That Counts as 1 Cup in the Milk Group	*Common Portions and Cup Equivalents*
Milk (Choose fat-free or low-fat milk most often.)	1 cup 1 half-pint container ½ cup evaporated milk	
Yogurt (Choose fat-free or low-fat yogurt most often.)	1 regular container (8 fl. oz.) 1 cup	1 small container (6 oz.) = ¾ cup 1 snack-size container (4 oz.) = ½ cup
Cheese (Choose low-fat cheeses most often.)	1½ oz. hard cheese (cheddar, mozzarella, Swiss, Parmesan) ⅓ cup shredded cheese 2 oz. processed cheese (American) ½ cup ricotta cheese 2 cups cottage cheese	1 slice hard cheese is equivalent to ½ cup milk 1 slice processed cheese is equivalent to ⅓ cup milk ½ cup cottage cheese is equivalent to ¼ cup milk
Milk-based desserts (Choose fat-free or low-fat types most often.)	1 cup pudding made with milk 1 cup frozen yogurt 1½ cups ice cream	1 scoop ice cream is equivalent to ⅓ cup milk

Beware of Calories

Unless your dairy products are low-fat or nonfat, the fat portion will count as discretionary calories. *(See pages 132–133 in Chapter 5.) When dairy products are sweetened, the added sugars also will count as discretionary calories. (See page 136 in Chapter 5.)*

Tips: Working Low-Fat Dairy Products into Your Diet

As some of the most versatile foods there are, dairy products are easy to work into your diet. The trick is in forgoing the whole-milk and high-fat versions.

▲ Gradually wean yourself from whole milk, switching first to reduced-fat (2 percent), then to low-fat (1 percent).

▲ Make a strong but short cup of coffee or tea, then add a half cup of heated low-fat or nonfat milk to make a whole cup.

▲ Drink low-fat or nonfat milk with meals.

▲ Substitute low-fat or nonfat milk on cereals.

▲ Make oatmeal and other hot cereal using low-fat or nonfat milk instead of water.

▲ Add low-fat or nonfat yogurt to smoothies.

▲ Use low-fat or nonfat milk for sauces and soups.

▲ Use low-fat or nonfat yogurt for dips, seasoned with herbs, garlic, and onions.

▲ Make low-fat or nonfat custard and puddings for desserts.

▲ Top fruit or other desserts with low-fat or nonfat yogurt.

▲ Use low-fat cheese in casseroles and pasta dishes.

▲ Opt for low-fat yogurt as a substitute for sour cream.

Shopping Tips

Don't make assumptions about the amount of calcium in specific foods. The amount of calcium in milk, whether skim or whole, is generally the same per serving, whereas the amount of calcium in the same size yogurt container (8 ounces) can vary by as much as 50 percent. Always check the label for calcium content.

Food labels are marked with a Percent Daily Value (% DV) for calcium (and other nutrients), which indicates what percentage of the Recommended Daily Allowances the product supplies. (See page 152 in Chapter 7.) Experts advise adult consumers to consume 1,000 milligrams of calcium in a daily 2,000-calorie diet. Adolescents, especially girls, require 1,300 milligrams, and postmenopausal women should consume 1,200 milligrams of calcium

Safety Tips

▲ *Chill perishable dairy products promptly. Discard food that has been left at temperatures between 40 and 140° F for more than two hours, even if it smells okay.*

▲ *Raw milk is a source of nutrients including beneficial bacteria such as* Lactobacillus acidophilus, *vitamins and enzymes, and calcium. But because it contains living organisms, it spoils quickly. The My Pyramid website recommends avoiding raw milk.*

▲ *Keep raw, cooked, and ready-to-eat foods separate.*

daily. Therefore, adults need 100% DV, teenagers need 130% DV, and postmenopausal women need 120% DV.

The Meat and Beans Group

My Pyramid Directive: Generally, adult women should consume five portions (1-ounce equivalents) of meat, poultry, fish, or beans per day. Adult men should consume six portions daily. This allotment varies slightly according to gender, age, and activity level. Toddlers require only one portion of this group daily, a requirement that grows as they mature.

Careful: *A portion of meat is only 1 ounce, usually about a cubic inch.*

What Is the Meat and Beans Group?

On the My Pyramid graphic, the slim purple segment on the far right is the Meat and Beans Group. It looks as if the USDA is trying to coax carnivores away from the meat counters. This pyramid's proportion of protein is even smaller than its counterpart on the previous Food Pyramid, a reflection of growing evidence that most Americans eat more animal protein than they need—and more than is good for them. Yes, we still require protein, but not as much animal protein as most people consume. Furthermore, the animal protein we eat needs to be a lot leaner.

My Pyramid calls this group Meat and Beans, but it actually includes many lean high-protein foods. These include the following.

Meats

Lean cuts of:

Beef

Ham

Lamb

Pork

Veal

Game meats:

Bison

Rabbit

Venison

Lean ground meats:

Beef

Pork

Lamb

Lean luncheon meats

Organ meats:

Liver

Giblets

Poultry

Chicken

Duck

Goose

Turkey

Ground chicken and turkey

Rabbit

Game hens and other game birds

Eggs

Chicken eggs

Duck eggs

Fish

Finfish such as:

Catfish

Cod

Flounder

Haddock

Halibut

Herring

Mackerel

Pollock

Porgy

Salmon

Sea bass

Snapper

Swordfish

Trout

Tuna

Shellfish such as:

Clams

Crab

Crayfish

Lobster

Mussels

Octopus

Oysters

Scallops

Squid (calamari)

Shrimp

Canned fish such as:
Anchovies
Clams
Tuna
Sardines

Beans and Peas (Legumes)

Black beans
Black-eyed peas
Chickpeas (garbanzo beans)
Kidney beans
Lentils
Lima beans (mature)
Mung beans
Navy beans
Pinto beans
Soybeans
Split peas
Tofu (bean curd made from soybeans)
White beans
Adzuki beans (also called aduki and azuki beans)
Great northern beans

Bean burgers:
Garden burgers
Veggie burgers
Falafel

Tempeh
Texturized vegetable protein (TVP)

Nuts and Seeds

Almonds

Cashews

Hazelnuts (filberts)

Mixed nuts

Peanuts

Peanut butter

Pecans

Pistachios

Pumpkinseeds

Sesame seeds

Sunflower seeds

Walnuts

Pine nuts

What do a split pea and a clam have in common? Essential amino acids, or EAAs, that's what. The human body, which is about 20 percent protein, relies on twenty-two amino acids as building blocks, only fourteen of which it manufactures on its own. We must acquire the remaining eight—*tryptophan, leucine, isoleucine, lysine, valine, threonine, phenylalanine,* and *methionine*—by eating protein. All the foods in the Meat and Beans Group deliver essential amino acids. Note that the foods are either "flesh" foods or the reproductive part of plants. This is why they are high in protein.

Research proves what vegetarians have railed about for years: that we can meet our protein requirement without burgers and drumsticks. Factors other than protein quality affect the desirability of one protein over another. Low-fat proteins are terrific, representing the wide end of the purple portion of the pyramid. Others, like fried chicken, are less so, as the narrow point of the pyramid symbolizes. One of meat's biggest drawbacks is its saturated fat. Therefore, My Pyramid drives home the message of lean choices and low-fat preparation. Substituting fish and beans for meat and poultry, by decreasing saturated fat intake, can lower cholesterol.

Why Is the Meats and Beans Group Important?

Foods in the meat, poultry, fish, eggs, and nuts and seeds group are vital for body health and maintenance, for the reasons that follow. However, choosing foods that are high in saturated fat and cholesterol from this group may undermine their positive effects, not just by attacking your good health, but also by adding extra calories. Be sure to prioritize lean selections.

Protein

Proteins, as mentioned, are the building blocks of all organic matter. Carbohydrates, fat, and protein all contain oxygen, hydrogen, and carbon, but only protein contains nitrogen, sulfur, and phosphorous. All of these are critical to life, for growth and maintenance. Protein in the blood balances water content, as well as acidity/alkalinity. Protein also combats infection by contributing to antibody formation. Our bone structure, teeth, nails, hair, tendons, and muscles are composed of fibrous proteins. To maintain them, we must eat adequate protein; otherwise, the body is obliged to borrow protein from its stores, depleting bones and muscles.

Amino Acid Content of Foods

	Food Group		
	(mg/g protein in 100 g of food)		
Amino acid	*Animal*	*Legumes*	*Nuts/Seeds*
Isoleucine	46.7 (4.7)	45.3 (4.2)	42.8 (6.1)
Leucine	79.6 (6.0)	78.9 (4.2)	73.5 (9.0)
Lysine	84.3 (7.1)	67.1 (3.8)	43.5 (12.7)

	Food Group *(mg/g protein in 100 g of food)*		
Amino acid	*Animal*	*Legumes*	*Nuts/Seeds*
Methionine	37.7 (3.3)	25.3 (2.8)	37.7 (11.7)
Phenylalanine	74.9 (8.2)	84.9 (6.3)	88.0 (16.9)
Threonine	43.4 (2.6)	40.0 (3.3)	37.9 (5.4)
Tryptophan	11.4 (1.5)	12.3 (2.4)	15.4 (4.6)
Valine	51.2 (5.6)	50.5 (4.0)	55.6 (10.3)

Vitamins

The *B vitamins—niacin, thiamin, riboflavin,* and *B_6*—help the body release energy and build new tissues, aid in the formation of red blood cells, and keep the nervous system functioning optimally. As an antioxidant, *vitamin E* helps buffer vitamin A and essential fatty acids from cell oxidation. Seeds are particularly good sources of vitamin E.

Minerals

Every body cell contains *iron,* most of it in combination with protein. Iron functions primarily as a carrier of oxygen in the blood. It is stored in the liver, spleen, and bone marrow. It contributes to protein metabolism and energy production. When iron is depleted, blood carries less oxygen to tissues, resulting in iron-deficiency anemia and decreased resistance to infections. *Zinc* supports biochemical reactions and boosts immune-system function. *Magnesium* works with calcium to build bones and release energy from muscles.

Fatty Acids

Our bodies demand *unsaturated fats* (more about this in the discussion of the Oils Group later in this chapter); however, they cannot manufacture them on their own. Therefore, we rely on monounsaturated fats and polyunsaturated fats in our diets to fill these gaps. Meat and poultry are *not* good sources, but fish, nuts, and seeds are. *Omega-3 fatty acids*—a type of polyunsaturated fat—are abundant in salmon, trout, herring, and several other cold-water fish.

How Much Meat and/or How Many Beans Should You Eat Daily?

Most of us eat plenty, if not too much, meat—too little of it lean—and inadequate fish, legumes, nuts, and seeds. The first step is figuring out how much from this food group you should be eating. The second step is determining how best to diversify and incorporate nonmeat proteins, and how to make most of the meat lean.

Look at the following chart. These are the minimum daily recommendations, for people who get *less* than thirty minutes of moderate physical activity a day. More-active people will require more. My Pyramid recommends at least thirty minutes of moderate exercise daily, as part of a healthy regime.

	Daily Recommendation	
Children	2–3 years old	2 oz. eq.
	4–8 years old	3–4 oz. eq.
Girls	9–13 years old	5 oz. eq.
	14–18 years old	5 oz. eq.
Boys	9–13 years old	5 oz. eq.
	14–18 years old	6 oz. eq.
Women	19–30 years old	5½ oz. eq.
	31–50 years old	5 oz. eq.
	51+ years old	5 oz. eq.
Men	19–30 years old	6½ oz. eq.
	31–50 years old	6 oz. eq.
	51+ years old	5½ oz. eq.

What Is an Ounce Equivalent?

Ounce equivalent *is My Pyramid's way of quantifying its meat and legume serving size recommendations. The word* serving *was used in the previous Food Pyramid. It was a tricky term because no one seemed to know exactly how much constituted a serving. My Pyramid tries to be more precise with its ounce equivalent.*

The term ounce equivalent *is based on the cooked measurement of the portion of any given food. Instead of saying* ounce, *it says* ounce equivalent. *See the following chart for help. To guess how many equivalents there might be in a food item that is not on the list, you always need to think in terms of the weight of the cooked food.*

How Much Equals a Meat and/or Beans Portion?

In general, 1 ounce of meat, ½ ounce of nuts or seeds, and ¼ cup uncooked legumes equal a 1 ounce equivalent from the Meat and Beans Group.

	Amount That Counts as 1 Ounce Equivalent in the Meat and Beans Group	*Common Portions and Ounce Equivalents*
Meats	1 oz. cooked lean beef	1 small steak (eye of round, filet) = 3½–4 oz. eq.

	1 oz. cooked lean pork or ham	1 small lean hamburger = 2–3 oz. eq.
Poultry	1 oz. cooked chicken or turkey, without skin	1 small chicken breast half = 3 oz. eq.
	1 sandwich slice of turkey (4½ × 2½ × ⅛″)	½ Cornish game hen = 4 oz. eq.
Fish	1 oz. cooked fish or shellfish	1 can of tuna, drained = 3–4 oz. eq.
	1 salmon steak = 4–6 oz. eq.	
	1 small trout = 3 oz. eq.	
Eggs	1 egg	
Nuts and seeds	½ oz. nuts (12 almonds, 24 pistachios, 7 walnut halves)	1 oz. of nuts or seeds = 2 oz. eq.
	½ oz. seeds (pumpkin, sunflower, or squash seeds, hulled, roasted)	
	1 Tbsp. peanut butter or almond butter	
Dry beans and peas	¼ cup cooked dry beans (black, kidney, pinto, or white beans)	1 cup split pea soup = 2 oz. eq.
		1 cup lentil soup = 2 oz. eq.
	¼ cup cooked dry peas	1 cup bean soup = 2 oz. eq.
	(chickpeas, cowpeas, lentils, or split peas)	
	¼ cup of baked beans refried beans	
	¼ cup (about 2 oz.) tofu	1 soy or bean burger patty = 2 oz. eq.
	1 oz. tempeh, cooked	
	¼ cup roasted soybeans	
	1 falafel patty (2¼″, 4 oz.)	
	2 Tbsp. hummus	

Tips: Working Those Lean Protein Foods into Your Diet

Americans rely on protein from fast food and processed food because it is quick and easy, but it is leaving us fat, malnourished, and disease prone. To reclaim our health, we must kick the habit. This takes not just commitment, but planning. By the time you get the hang of preparing and eating lean, you will begin to look and feel better.

Chances are, you will also cultivate a more sophisticated palate. Since My Pyramid recommends that only about one-tenth of your total diet be composed of protein foods, an amount far smaller than many Americans eat, you can immediately shift from drive-through dining to grazing on nuts and seeds. By weaning yourself from big meat portions and trading beef for nuts and poultry for legumes, you might even save money.

A lot of the shift is mental. Many Americans are accustomed to thinking of the meat, poultry, or fish portion of a meal as the main attraction. After all, the square meal is an American tradition, even though it is making us sick and in some cases killing us. Yet in healthier-eating cultures, most of every meal is carbohydrates and vegetables, with a few morsels of animal product thrown in.

We are lucky in the United States to have many immigrant cultures to broaden our dietary horizons. On the My Pyramid regime, you need not sit down to a lonely baked potato and salad with no meat. Instead, you can enjoy lamb curry with rice and lentils, or chard-stuffed cannelloni with walnut sauce, or chicken cassoulet with white beans, chicken, and ham, or Thai salmon rolls with peanut sauce. Take time to learn about and come up with similar appealing and nourishing combinations.

Remember that the daily allotment of protein is about the same size as a cube and a half of butter. That 2 inches by

2 inches by 3 inches is a whole lot smaller than a T-bone steak and can be spread out over the whole day.

Any ethnic food immediately inspires wholly palatable ideas:

▲ Italian pasta, gnocchi, or polenta with braised fish, poultry, lamb, pork, beef, or toasted nuts

▲ French composé salads with slices of grilled meat, vegetables, and savory dressing

▲ Spanish paella with seasoned rice, seafood, and chicken

▲ Japanese sushi

▲ Greek stuffed eggplant

▲ Armenian tabouli with lamb kebabs

▲ Moroccan couscous with chicken and vegetables

▲ Indian curries with rice, *dahl* (bean dish), and pungent meats

▲ Thai dishes of spicy meats and vegetables with rice

▲ Chinese stir-fries

▲ Mexican enchiladas, burritos, or tacos

Guiding Principles

▲ Make sure you get adequate quantities of all essential amino acids by varying the protein foods you eat.

▲ Choose fish frequently, particularly fish rich in omega-3 fatty acids (salmon, trout, and herring).

▲ Make dry beans or peas the main dish more often.

▲ Incorporate nuts and seeds, as well as nut and seed butters, into sandwiches, sauces, salads, snacks, and main dishes. Think slivered almonds on vegetables, cashews instead of beef in stir-fry, toasted walnuts on a green salad, pine nuts in pesto pasta, and ground pecans on low-fat ice cream or yogurt.

Maximize Protein Utilization with Combinations

Variety is one way to make sure we get sufficient protein, in the form of the essential amino acids. Another way is to eat some meat, poultry, and fish every day. The third way, which many vegetarians subscribe to, is to combine whole grains with beans or seeds. Here are some examples of combinations that augment the protein utilization of nonmeat foods:

▲ *Millet + adzuki beans*

▲ *Brown rice + sunflower seeds*

▲ *Soybeans + rice*

▲ *Soybeans + sesame, corn, wheat, or rye*

▲ *Peanuts + grain or coconut*

▲ *Grain + beans or leafy greens*

▲ *Beans + corn or rice*

▲ *Peas + wheat*[26]

What Is Healthful Preparation?

Shop Lean

Buy the following cuts of meat:

▲ Beef roasts and steaks: round-eye, top round, bottom round, round tip, top loin, top sirloin, chuck shoulder roast, chuck arm roast, 90 percent lean hamburger

▲ Veal: all cuts except ground veal

▲ Pork roasts and chops: tenderloin, center loin, ham

▲ Lamb and mutton roasts and chops: leg, loin, fore shanks

▲ Chicken, turkey, and other poultry: light and dark meat, without the skin

▲ Lean and low-fat luncheon meats: lean roast beef, turkey, ham

▲ Fish and shellfish: all, except when canned or marinated in oil

Avoid the following:

▲ High- or medium-fat ground beef

▲ Beef and pork sausage, hot dogs, bacon, bologna, salami

▲ Liver

▲ Domestic duck

▲ More than one egg yolk per egg dish

▲ Excessive nuts and seeds, since they are high in fat

Cook Lean

▲ Trim away all the fat you can see, before cooking.

▲ Broil, roast, grill, or poach food instead of frying.

▲ Use no-stick pans and healthful cooking oils (see pages 113–114).

▲ Drain off any fat that appears during cooking.

▲ Skip or limit breading on meat, poultry, and fish dishes. (Breading soaks up fat and adds extra calories.)

▲ Prepare low-fat or no-fat sauces.

Read Labels

Foods high in saturated fat, trans fat, and cholesterol can elevate "bad" cholesterol, as reflected in higher levels of low-density lipoprotein (LDL). (See more about this in the Oils Group section later in this chapter). Lower-fat versions are available. Check packaged and processed food labels, and choose products with fewer of these unhealthy ingredients.

Too much salt (sodium chloride) can lead to hypertension. Processed meats such as ham, sausage, hot dogs or frankfurters, and luncheon or deli meats have added sodium. Check product labels and avoid those that say "self-basting" or "contains up to % of _____ (a sodium-containing solution).

Safety Tips

Our bodies accommodate some bacteria and even use them to thrive. Just like us, meat, poultry, fish, and eggs contain bacteria. Processing can kill some bacteria and introduce others that may not be healthy for humans to ingest. Usually, it is unhealthy to eat animal foods without cooking them first, which kills the bacteria. Similarly, leaving food unrefrigerated or at a tepid temperature for a period of time encourages bacteria to grow. Therefore, the following procedures are very important.

▲ Separate raw, cooked, and ready-to-eat foods.

▲ Do not wash or rinse meat or poultry because handling could cause the spread of salmonella bacteria. Wash hands after handling meat.

▲ Wash cutting boards, knives, utensils, and countertops in hot, soapy water after preparing each food item and before going on to the next one.

▲ Store raw meat, poultry, and seafood on the bottom shelf of the refrigerator so juices do not drip onto other foods.

▲ Cook foods to a safe temperature to kill microorganisms. Use a meat thermometer, which measures the internal temperature of cooked meat and poultry, to make sure that the meat is cooked all the way through.

▲ Chill (refrigerate) perishable food promptly and defrost food properly. Refrigerate or freeze perishables, prepared food, and leftovers within two hours.

▲ Plan ahead to defrost food. Never defrost food on the kitchen counter at room temperature. Thaw food by placing it in the refrigerator, submerging airtight packaged food in cold tap water, or defrosting on a plate in the microwave.

▲ Avoid raw or partially cooked eggs and foods containing raw eggs and raw or undercooked meat and poultry.

▲ Women who may become pregnant, pregnant women, nursing mothers, and young children should avoid some types of fish and eat types lower in mercury. See www.cfsan.fda.gov/~dms/admehg3.html or call 1-888-SAFEFOOD for more information.

Healthy Protein Tips for Children

Loading up on candy keeps children revved up, and greasy foods give them a feeling of fullness. One of the reasons American children so crave sugar, fats, and salt is that despite the quantities of food they eat, they are poorly nourished. It is up to families to establish good eating habits and send them off to school properly nourished. Children usually love meat, beans, and nut butters. The other nonprotein food items are the problem.

▲ Substitute low-fat ham and an egg, or oatmeal with soy milk and fruit, for sugary cereals at breakfast.

▲ Hearty soups and nut-butter sandwiches are much better lunch fare than high-fat lunch meats.

▲ For fast food, order fish tacos instead of burgers.

▲ On pizzas, substitute chicken or shrimp for pepperoni.

▲ Teach your children about other cultures so they will be curious about eating new foods.

▲ Lobby your school district to improve school lunches.

▲ Get your children to help you convert to meals based on complex carbohydrates by shopping and preparing food together.

Meeting Requirements in Vegetarian Diets

Just like meat eaters, vegetarians need to consume a variety of foods and the right amount of foods to meet calorie and nutrient requirements. Nutrients that may challenge vegetarians are those that are readily available in meat: protein, iron, calcium, zinc, and vitamin B_{12}. Following are guidelines to help vegetarians make sure they get the necessary quota:

▲ *Protein* needs can easily be met by eating a variety of plant-based foods. Sources of protein for vegetarians include beans, nuts, nut butters, peas, and soy products (tofu, tempeh, veggie burgers). Milk products and eggs are also good protein sources for lacto-ovo vegetarians.

▲ *Iron* sources include iron-fortified breakfast cereals, spinach, kidney beans, black-eyed peas, lentils, turnip greens, molasses, whole-wheat breads, peas, and some dried fruits (dried apricots, prunes, raisins).

▲ *Calcium* sources include fortified breakfast cereals, soy products (tofu, soy-based beverages), calcium-fortified orange juice, and some dark green leafy vegetables (collard greens, turnip greens, bok choy, mustard greens). Milk products are excellent calcium sources for lacto vegetarians.

▲ *Zinc* sources include many types of beans (white beans, kidney beans, and chickpeas), zinc-fortified breakfast cereals, wheat germ, and pumpkinseeds.

▲ *Vitamin B_{12}* is found in animal products and some fortified foods. Sources of vitamin B_{12} for vegetarians include milk products, eggs, and foods that have been fortified with vitamin B_{12}. These include breakfast cereals, soy-based beverages, veggie burgers, and nutritional yeast.

The absence of meat does not prevent creativity and gusto. It promotes it! It is a mistake to think of vegetarianism as second best to eating animals and animal products. Get yourself some really good vegetarian cookbooks (see the resource list at the back of this book). Build meals around protein sources that are naturally low in fat, such as beans, lentils, and rice. Do not overload meals with high-fat cheeses to replace the meat.

▲ Calcium-fortified soy-based beverages can provide calcium in amounts similar to milk. They are usually low in fat and do not contain cholesterol.

▲ Transform foods that typically contain meat, poultry, or fish into vegetarian dishes. You will increase vegetable intake and cut saturated fat and cholesterol. Consider:
  ▲ Pasta primavera or pasta with marinara or pesto sauce
  ▲ Veggie pizza
  ▲ Vegetable lasagna
  ▲ Tofu-vegetable stir-fry
  ▲ Vegetable lo mein
  ▲ Vegetable kebabs
  ▲ Bean burritos or tacos

Vegetarian products that look (and may taste) like their nonvegetarian counterparts usually have lower saturated fat and contain no cholesterol.

▲ For breakfast, try soy-based sausage patties or links.

▲ Rather than hamburgers, try veggie burgers. A variety of kinds are available, made with soybeans, vegetables, and/or rice.

▲ Add vegetarian meat substitutes to soups and stews to boost protein without adding saturated fat or cholesterol. These include tempeh (cultured soybeans with a chewy texture), tofu, and wheat gluten (seitan).

▲ For barbecues, try veggie or garden burgers, soy hot dogs, marinated tofu or tempeh, and veggie kebabs.

▲ Make bean burgers, lentil burgers, or pita halves with falafel (spicy ground chickpea patties).

Usually, but not always, faux flesh foods are very different from meat, poultry, and fish and will disappoint consumers who hope not to notice the difference. People who still long for meat will wind up scoffing at "can't believe it's not meat" claims. By contrast, those who embrace vegetarianism with the desire to create a non-animal-based cuisine that is exceptional on its own merits will find much to lure them.

Most restaurants can accommodate vegetarian modifications to menu items by substituting meatless sauces, omitting meat from stir-fries, and adding vegetables or pasta in place of meat. These substitutions are more likely to be available at restaurants that make food to order. Some restaurants offer soy options (texturized vegetable protein) as a substitute for meat, and soy cheese as a substitute for regular cheese.

The Oils Group

My Pyramid Directive: **Most diets contain more than the minimum requirement for oil. Generally, adult women should consume 5 to 6 teaspoons of monounsaturated and/or polyunsaturated oil per day. Adult men should consume 6 to 7 teaspoons per day. This allotment varies slightly according to gender, age, and activity level. Toddlers require only 3 to 4 teaspoons, a requirement that grows as they mature.**

What Is the Oils Group?

On the My Pyramid graphic, the thin yellow segment to the right of the red Fruit Group represents the Oils Group. The Oils Group prioritizes healthy oils and discourages fats that are less beneficial and may even lead to health problems. Healthy oils are fats that are liquid at room temperature. Used sparingly (but not eliminated altogether), these vegetable oils provide nutrients and help us absorb other nutrients. Foods high in healthy oils are

▲ Seeds and nuts, including avocados

▲ Olives

▲ Cold-water fish

▲ Extra-virgin olive oil

▲ Mayonnaise with no trans fat

▲ Salad dressing with no trans fat

▲ Soft margarine with no trans fat (tub or squeeze)

Animal-derived fats contain cholesterol. No vegetable oils contain cholesterol. That is why salad dressings and cooking oils are invariably described as "low cholesterol."

The Four Oil Categories

These categories are organized in order of desirability. The last two categories, saturated fats and trans fats, are less healthy.

High in Monounsaturated Fats

These are the most healthy oils.

▲ Extra-virgin olive oil

▲ Canola oil (rapeseed oil)

▲ Almond oil

▲ Flaxseed oil

▲ Hazelnut oil

Monounsaturated fats are liquid at room temperature. The healthiest oils, they are abundant in some vegetable oils. By raising HDL (good) cholesterol and lowering LDL (bad) cholesterol levels, they may lower total blood cholesterol levels.

High in Polyunsaturated Fats

▲ Sunflower oil

▲ Safflower oil

▲ Soybean oil

▲ Corn oil

▲ Cottonseed oil

▲ Peanut oil

▲ Sesame oil

▲ Walnut oil

Polyunsaturated fats are liquid at room temperature and can be found in vegetable oils. They spoil easily at room temperature and should be stored in the refrigerator or (if you will be using them quickly) in the dark. They are thought to lower both good and bad cholesterol. (See "Cholesterol" box on page 116.) Polyunsaturated fats contain some fatty acids that are necessary for health—hence, they are called *essential fatty acids*. (More about this in a moment.)

High in Saturated Fats

Eat these only occasionally or not at all.

▲ Butter.

▲ Beef, lamb, pork, and chicken fat.

▲ Lard.

▲ Tallow or suet.

▲ Coconut oil and palm kernel oil, though liquid, are considered solid fats and should be avoided; they are high in saturated fats, which are unhealthy.

Saturated fats are solid at room temperature. They come from animals and tropical oils. Coconut oil and palm oil are two saturated vegetable oils. Saturated fats do not go rancid as easily as unsaturated fats. They may cause the total blood cholesterol level to rise. (Note: Benefits are associated with coconut oil.)

High in Trans Fats

Growing awareness of the hazards of trans fats has manufacturers scrambling to remove them from their products. Foods made with trans fats are required to be so labeled. It is up to consumers to watch out for them. Here are some foods that may have trans fats:

▲ Shortening

▲ Stick margarine

▲ Baked goods

▲ Icings

▲ Fried foods

▲ Spreads

▲ Microwave popcorn

> *Important: Health experts recommend that you keep your intake of saturated fat, trans fat, and cholesterol as low as possible as part of a nutritionally balanced diet.*

Trans fats are made when manufacturers add hydrogen to vegetable oil, in the presence of small amounts of metals. This process is known as *partial hydrogenation*. Partially hydrogenated vegetable oils are much less expensive than the fats originally favored by bakers, such as butter or lard. The shelf life and flavor stability of foods containing trans fats are greater, too. Snack foods, fried foods, baked goods, salad dressings, and other processed foods are therefore apt to contain trans fats, as are vegetable shortenings and margarine. Research has proven that trans fats are difficult to digest and can increase the possibility of cardiovascular disease.

Cholesterol

Cholesterol is a soft, waxy substance found among the lipids (fats) in the bloodstream and in every cell. Our bodies use cholesterol to form cell membranes and some hormones. Too much cholesterol in the blood, however, may lead to coronary heart disease and/or strokes.

Cholesterol does not dissolve in the blood, but is carried to and from the cells by special carriers called lipoproteins. Low-density lipoproteins (LDLs) are the major cholesterol carriers in the blood. If too much LDL cholesterol circulates in the blood, it can slowly build up in the arteries feeding the heart and brain, forming plaque that clogs those arteries.

High-density lipoproteins (HDLs) carry cholesterol away from the arteries and back to the liver, where it is passed from the body. HDL cholesterol is known as "good" cholesterol because a high HDL level seems to protect against heart attacks. Exposure to smoke and other toxins appears to lower HDL levels.

People get cholesterol in two ways. The body—mainly the liver—produces cholesterol. The rest comes from eating animals that contain it. Eating saturated fatty acids raises blood cholesterol. So does trans fat. You should limit your average daily cholesterol intake to under 300 milligrams, or less if you have high blood cholesterol.

Why Are Beneficial Oils from the Oils Group Important?

Overall Health

Judicious use of oils high in monounsaturated and polyunsaturated fats reduces the risk of

▲ Stroke, coronary heart disease, and other cardiovascular diseases

▲ Certain cancers, such as mouth, stomach, and colorectal cancer

▲ Bone disease

▲ High blood pressure

It improves

▲ Cellular function

▲ Bones, skin, hair, and eyes

▲ Immunity

▲ Cold and heat tolerance[27]

Eating prudently from the beneficial Oils Group—the polyunsaturated and monunsaturated fats—fulfills these vital nutritional roles in the following ways:

▲ Unsaturated fats provide a ready energy source, with an immediate supply of calories to fuel our activities and body functions.

▲ Unsaturated fats protect organs from trauma and cold, keeping internal temperature consistent and minimizing temperature-related stress.

▲ Cell membranes are composed of *phospholipids,* or fatty acids. The fluidity of the cell membranes keeps messages flowing to and from the cells efficiently. Unsaturated fats permit greater cell membrane flexibility and permeability.

▲ Unsaturated fats encourage positive gene expression, mean-
ing that they activate genes that minimize the risk of disease.[28]

▲ Vitamins A, D, E, and K—found in the fat component of
both vegetables and animal foods—are critical, and they cannot be absorbed except in the presence of fat. Alcohol somewhat diminishes the absorption of fat-soluble vitamins.
When vitamin D is absorbed, calcium can be utilized. Vitamins A and E are important antioxidants and boost immunity. The Milk Group section includes a discussion of
vitamin D's benefits to our bones and teeth. Vitamin K is
necessary for blood clotting.

▲ Unsaturated fat provides some protection against heart disease and high cholesterol. Researchers have correlated the
lower rate of heart disease in the Mediterranean region to the
quantities of olive oil used in Mediterranean cooking. Sure
enough, extra-virgin olive oil, rich in monounsaturated fats,
increases high-density lipoproteins, counterbalancing the bad
cholesterol, low-density lipoproteins. The result is a lower
overall blood cholesterol level.

In addition to calling attention to unsaturated fats and
their recommended proportions, My Pyramid educates us
about the preponderance of unhealthy fats in American diets.
Diets high in saturated and trans fat (hydrogenated vegetable
oils) often lead to plaque-clogged arteries (atherosclerosis).
They raise cholesterol, which further exacerbates the stress on
the vascular system and leads to high blood pressure. Four very
common cancers—of the colon and rectum, the ovaries, the
prostate, and the breast—are associated with a high-fat, low-
fiber diet, and particularly with saturated fats found in animal
foods.

Therefore, the task is to balance oil intake. My Pyramid
suggests that we decrease the saturated fats and increase the
polyunsaturated and monounsaturated fats. It comes down to

using all fats and oils sparingly, with a preference for olive oil and other monounsaturated fats.

Essential Fatty Acids

Essential fatty acids (omega-3 and omega-6) support the cardiovascular, nervous, reproductive, and immune systems. Essential fatty acids can reduce cholesterol levels and the risk of heart disease. They are important for normal growth of the blood vessels and nerves. They also help lubricate the skin and other tissues.

Oil Foods High in Omega-3 Essential Fatty Acids

Flaxseed and flaxseed oil

Soybean products and soybean oil

Canola (rapeseed) oil

Pumpkinseeds

Walnuts and walnut oil

Cold-water fish (salmon, herring, cod, bluefish, tuna, mackerel, shrimp, flounder)

Oil Foods High in Omega-6 Essential Fatty Acids

Soybean products and soybean oil

Safflower oil

Sunflower seeds and sunflower oil

Corn and corn oil

Sesame seeds and sesame oil

Wheat germ

Olive Oil

How Much Oil Should You Eat Daily?

Although consuming some oil is necessary to stay healthy, oils still contain calories. In fact, both oils and solid fats contain about 120 calories per tablespoon. Furthermore, fat is present in many protein and carbohydrate foods. My Pyramid recommends that no more than 25 percent of our total caloric intake should be fat-derived. (Americans' average caloric intake is presently up to 40 percent from fat.) *The amount of oil My Pyramid recommends is approximately one-tenth that consumed by the average American.* Therefore, we need to cut back on oil to balance total calorie intake, and choose beneficial oils as often as possible. Nutrition Facts labels provide information to help you make smart choices (see Chapter 7).

Maximum recommended total daily amounts for people who get *less* than thirty minutes per day of moderate physical activity are shown in the following chart. My Pyramid recommends at least thirty minutes of moderate exercise daily, as part of a healthy regime. Those who are more physically active may be able to consume more while staying within calorie needs.

*Daily Allowance**

Children	2–3 years old	3 tsp.
	4–8 years old	4 tsp.
Girls	9–13 years old	5 tsp.
	14–18 years old	5 tsp.
Boys	9–13 years old	5 tsp.
	14–18 years old	6 tsp.
Women	19–30 years old	6 tsp.
	31–50 years old	5 tsp.
	51+ years old	5 tsp.
Men	19–30 years old	7 tsp.
	31–50 years old	6 tsp.
	51+ years old	6 tsp.

How Many Calories Are in Beneficial-Oil Foods?

The following chart serves as a quick guide to the calories found in some common beneficial-oil foods.

	Amount of Food	*Amount of Oil, Tsp./g*	*Calories from Oil (approximate)*	*Total Calories (approximate)*
Oils:				
Vegetable oils (such as canola, corn, cottonseed, olive, peanut, safflower, soybean, and sunflower)	1 Tbsp.	3 tsp/14 g	120	120
Foods rich in oils:				
Margarine, soft (trans fat free)	1 Tbsp.	2½ tsp./11 g	100	100
Mayonnaise	1 Tbsp.	2½ tsp./11 g	100	100
Mayonnaise-type salad dressing	1 Tbsp.	1 tsp./5 g	45	55
Italian dressing	2 Tbsp.	2 tsp./8 g	75	85
Thousand Island dressing	2 Tbsp.	2½ tsp./11 g	100	120
Olives, ripe, canned	4 large	½ tsp./2 g	15	20
Avocado*	½ medium	3 tsp./15 g	130	160
Peanut butter*	2 Tbsp.	4 tsp./16 g	140	190
Peanuts, dry roasted*	1 oz.	3 tsp./14 g	120	165
Mixed nuts, dry roasted*	1 oz.	3 tsp./15 g	130	170
Cashews, dry roasted*	1 oz.	3 tsp./13 g	115	165
Almonds, dry roasted*	1 oz.	3 tsp./15 g	130	170
Hazelnuts*	1 oz.	4 tsp./18 g	160	185
Sunflower seeds*	1 oz.	3 tsp./14 g	120	165

*Avocados are part of the Fruit Group; nuts and seeds are part of the Meat and Beans Group.

Foods to Eat in Extreme Moderation

Total Fat, Saturated Fat, Trans Fat, and Cholesterol Content per Serving[29]

Product	Common Serving Size	Total Fat, g	Saturated Fat, g	%DV for Saturated Fat	Trans Fat, g	Combined Saturated and Trans Fat, g	Cholesterol, mg	%DV for Cholesterol
French-fried potatoes* (fast food)	Medium (147 g)	27	7	35%	8	15	0	0%
Butter[†]	1 Tbsp.	11	7	35%	0	7	30	10%
Margarine, stick[‡]	1 Tbsp.	11	2	10%	3	5	0	0%
Shortening*	1 Tbsp.	13	3.5	18%	4	7.5	0	0%
Potato chips*	Small bag (42.5 g)	11	2	10%	3	5	0	0%
Milk, whole*	1 cup	7	4.5	23%	0	4.5	35	12%
Doughnut*	1	18	4.5	23%	5	9.5	25	8%
Cookies* (cream-filled)	3 (30 g)	6	1	5%	2	3	0	0%
Candy bar*	1 (40 g)	10	4	20%	3	7	<5	1%
Cake, pound*	1 slice (80 g)	16	3.5	18%	4.5	8	0	0%

*1995 USDA Composition Data.

[†]Butter values from FDA Table of Trans Values, 1/30/95.

[‡]Values derived from 2002 USDA National Nutrient Database for Standard Reference, Release 15.

Heating Oil . . .

▲ DOES OXYGENIZE AND HYDROGENIZE OIL TO A
SMALL DEGREE, MAKING IT MORE SATURATED.

▲ DOES DIMINISH OIL'S NUTRITIONAL VALUE.

*The higher the heat and the longer food is fried, the
worse the effect on the oil. That is why it is best to steam
food first, then sauté it quickly at the last minute. Or you
can skip the sautéing entirely and just drizzle oil over the
cooked food. Olive oil remains stable at a higher temperature than other oils.*

Tips for Balancing Your Oil Intake in Preference of Beneficial Oils

▲ Keep olive oil, canola oil, and mayonnaise in your larder.

▲ Substitute flavorful olive oil for butter in recipes.

▲ Use olive oil and nut oils on bread instead of butter or margarine.

▲ Drizzle olive oil, instead of butter or margarine, over vegetables after they are cooked.

▲ Supplement your diet with flaxseed oil.

▲ Eat cold-water fish (salmon, herring, cod, bluefish, tuna,
mackerel, shrimp, flounder).

▲ Use tub margarine instead of stick margarine.

▲ Make quiche and savory tart dough with olive oil instead of
butter or shortening.

Now that you better understand My Pyramid's six food groups and have an idea of how much of each you should be eating, you can start right in, modifying what you eat to make sure you are more healthfully nourished. If you eat prudently, you will have leftover calories you can use for treats, as you will read in Chapter 5.

Meal Size

Most people eat too much. Some people eat too little. But almost everyone eats too little of the right thing. My Pyramid makes clear that the protein, fat, and sugar portions that Americans consume need downsizing. No more meat, poultry, or fish in an entire day than the size of your palm (minus the fingers). No more fat in an entire day than the size of two thumbs. That includes the butter or fats in baked goods. Clearly, some austerity measures are necessary. If you need more bulk or bigger meals than you are getting with these measures, you must compensate with whole grains, vegetables, and fruit. Otherwise, you may be putting your health at risk.

CHAPTER FIVE

Maximizing Your Bonus Calories

My Pyramid Directive: Eating the lowest-fat and less-sweetened foods in recommended portions from the six food groups leaves room for bonuses, called *discretionary calories*. These may be extra helpings from the six food groups, higher-fat foods, sweets, or alcohol. Their total calories, when added to the rest of your calorie intake, should not exceed the maximum calorie recommendation for your gender, age, and activity level.

What Are Discretionary Calories?

Eating recommended portions from My Pyramid's six food groups—Grains, Vegetables, Fruits, Milk, Meat and Beans, and Oils—will supply the nutrients you need to optimize your health. These nutrients are *essential*. If you eat sensibly, keeping your calorie intake as low as possible, you may find that you have not used up the amount of calories recommended for your gender, age, and activity level (see page 128). Those extra calories are called *discretionary calories.*

Discretionary calories are like a bonus. You can use them for dietary sprees, eating whatever you want, as long as adding them to the other calories you ingest does not make you exceed the amount of calories recommended for your gender, age, and activity level.

My Pyramid suggests thinking about calories as you do money. The recommended calories for your gender, age, and activity level are your budgetary allowance. This is the number of calories that keeps your body functioning and provides energy for physical activities.

With a financial budget, the essentials are items like shelter and food. In a calorie budget, the essentials are the calories required to supply necessary vitamins, minerals, fiber, and oils. If you want to purchase these nutrients at bargain-basement prices, you will select the lowest-fat and no-sugar-added forms of foods from each food group.

If you can keep your caloric intake to a minimum, you may be able to spend more calories than the amount required to meet your nutritional needs. These calories are the extras that can be used on luxuries like solid fats, added sugars, and alcohol, or on more food from any food group. They are your discretionary calories. In a financial budget these would correspond to things like extravagant clothes, movies, and vacations, which you can indulge in after your shelter and food needs have been met.

If, instead, you try to meet your nutritional requirements with high-fat, sweet foods, you will spend your entire budgetary allowance—and may even fail to get the nutrients you require. *This is the way most Americans eat.* Our citizens have weight and health problems because they blow their budgetary calorie allowance on foods that do not provide adequate nourishment first. Then, still feeling famished, they overspend the allowance with additional helpings and bigger portions of the wrong foods. If this were a financial budget, this society would be living with extravagant clothes, movies, and vacations, but without food and shelter.

How Many Discretionary Calories Can You Have?

The discretionary calories allowance is based on estimated calorie needs by age/sex group. Physical activity increases calorie needs, so those who are more physically active need more total calories and have a larger discretionary calorie allowance. *The discretionary calorie allowance is part of total estimated calorie needs, not in addition to total calorie needs.* The chart on page 128 can serve as a general guide.

As you can see, discretionary calorie allowances are miniscule, especially for those who are not physically active. For example, assume your calorie budget is 2,000 calories per day. Of

Some Spree Foods Are Unhealthy

Eating 150 calories' worth of whole yogurt is a healthy treat. Even 150 calories' worth of chocolate has some health benefits. By contrast, 150 calories of trans fat and synthetic-ingredient-filled snack foods may actually be harmful, particularly to people with certain medical conditions.

Age and Sex	Not Physically Active*		Physically Active†	
	Estimated total calorie need	Estimated discretionary calorie allowance	Estimated total calorie need	Estimated discretionary calorie allowance
Children 2–3 years old	1,000 calories	165‡	1,000–1,400 calories	165–170
Children 4–8 years old	1,200–1,400 calories	170‡	1,400–1,800 calories	170–195
Girls 9–13 years old	1,600 calories	130	1,600–2,200 calories	130–290
Boys 9–13 years old	1,800 calories	195	1,800–2,600 calories	195–410
Girls 14–18 years old	1,800 calories	195	2,000–2,400 calories	265–360
Boys 14–18 years old	2,200 calories	290	2,400–3,200 calories	360–650
Females 19–30 years old	2,000 calories	265	2,000–2,400 calories	265–360
Males 19–30 years old	2,400 calories	360	2,600–3,000 calories	410–510
Females 31–50 years old	1,800 calories	195	2,000–2,200 calories	265–290
Males 31–50 years old	2,200 calories	290	2,400–3,000 calories	360–510
Females 51+ years old	1,600 calories	130	1,800–2,200 calories	195–290
Males 51+ years old	2,000 calories	265	2,200–2,800 calories	290–425

*These amounts are appropriate for individuals who get less than thirty minutes of moderate physical activity most days.

†These amounts are appropriate for individuals who get at least thirty minutes (lower calorie level) to at least sixty minutes (higher calorie level) of moderate physical activity most days.

‡The number of discretionary calories is higher for children eight and younger than it is for older children or adults consuming the same number of calories, because younger children's nutrient needs are lower. Therefore, less food from the basic food groups and fewer essential calories are needed.

these calories, you will spend at least 1,735 calories for essential nutrients only if you choose foods without fat or added sugar. That leaves you 265 discretionary calories. Many people's discretionary calorie allowance is totally used by the foods they choose in each food group, such as higher-fat meats, cheeses, whole milk, or sweetened bakery products. Fats are concentrated sources of calories. Even small amounts of foods high in solid fats will use up the discretionary calorie allowance quickly. *A high percentage of Americans use up this allowance before lunchtime each day.*

Use your discretionary calorie allowance to

▲ Eat more foods from any food group that the food group guides recommend.

▲ Eat higher-calorie forms of foods—those that contain solid fats or added sugars. (More about these foods follows.)

▲ Add fats or sweeteners to foods. Examples are sauces, salad dressings, sugar, syrup, and butter.

▲ Eat or drink items that are mostly fats, caloric sweeteners, and/or alcohol, such as candy, soda, wine, and beer.

Counting the Discretionary Calories You Eat

The following chart provides a quick guide to the number of discretionary calories in foods commonly consumed by Americans every day. It does not include foods high in solid fats or added sugars (those follow in a few pages). To demonstrate how better choices help us save discretionary calories, the chart includes fat-free and low-fat foods.

Food	Amount	Estimated Total Calories	Estimated Discretionary Calories
Milk Group			
Fat-free milk	1 cup	85	0
1% milk	1 cup	100	20

Food	Amount	Estimated Total Calories	Estimated Discretionary Calories
2% milk (reduced fat)	1 cup	125	40
Whole milk	1 cup	145	65
Low-fat chocolate milk	1 cup	160	75
Cheddar cheese	1½ ounces	170	90
Nonfat mozzarella	1½ ounces	65	0
Whole-milk mozzarella	1½ ounces	130	45
Fruit-flavored low-fat yogurt	1 cup (8 fl. oz.)	240–250	100–115
Frozen yogurt	1 cup	220	140
Ice cream, vanilla	1 cup	290	205
Cheese sauce	¼ cup	120	75
Meat and Beans Group			
Extra-lean ground beef, 95% lean	3 oz., cooked	165	0
Regular ground beef, 80% lean	3 oz., cooked	230	65
Turkey roll, light meat	3 slices (1 oz. each)	125	0
Roasted chicken breast (skinless)	3 oz.	140	0
Roasted chicken thigh with skin	3 oz.	210	70
Fried chicken with skin and batter	3 wings	475	335
Beef sausage, precooked	3 oz., cooked	345	180
Pork sausage	3 oz., cooked	290	125
Beef bologna	3 slices (1 oz. each)	265	100
Grains			
Whole-wheat bread	1 slice (1 oz.)	70	0
White bread	1 slice (1 oz.)	70	0
English muffin	1 muffin	135	0
Blueberry muffin	1 small (2 oz.)	185	45
Croissant	1 medium (2 oz.)	230	95
Biscuit, plain	1–2.5″ diameter	130	60

Food	Amount	Estimated Total Calories	Estimated Discretionary Calories
Corn bread	1 piece (2½ × 2½ × 1¼")	190	50
Graham crackers	2 large pieces	120	50
Whole-wheat crackers	5 crackers	90	20
Round snack crackers	7 crackers	105	35
Chocolate chip cookies	2 large	135	70
Cake-type doughnuts, plain	2 mini doughnuts, 1½" diameter	120	50
Glazed doughnut, yeast type	1 medium, 3¾" diameter	240	165
Cinnamon sweet roll	1–3 oz. roll	310	100
Vegetables			
French fries	1 medium order	460	325
Onion rings	1 order (8–9 rings)	275	160
Extras*			
Regular soda	1 can (12 fl. oz.)	155	155
Regular soda	1 bottle (20 fl. oz.)	260	260
Diet soda	1 can (12 fl. oz.)	5	5
Fruit punch	1 cup	115	115
Table wine	5 fl. oz.	115	115
Beer (regular)	12 fl. oz.	145	145
Beer (light)	12 fl. oz.	110	110
Distilled spirits (80 proof)	1½ fl. oz.	95	95
Butter	1 tsp.	35	35
Stick margarine	1 tsp.	35	35
Cream cheese	1 Tbsp.	50	50
Heavy (whipping) cream	1 Tbsp.	50	50
Dessert topping, frozen, semisolid	1 Tbsp.	15	15
Gravy, canned	¼ cup	30	30

*All of the calories in candy, sodas, alcoholic beverages, and solid fats are discretionary calories because they do not supply nutrients that are not covered in other food groups.

Tip: The calories per serving are listed on the Nutrition Facts label on food packages. Be sure to compare the stated serving size to the amount actually eaten. If you eat twice the stated serving size, you will take in twice the calories.

Discretionary Calories from Solid Fats

Unlike the beneficial oils discussed in the Oils Group section of Chapter 4, solid fats are fats that are solid at room temperature, like butter and shortening. Solid fats come from many animal foods and can be made from vegetable oils through a process called *hydrogenation*.

Some common solid fats are

▲ Butter

▲ Beef fat (tallow, suet)

▲ Chicken fat

▲ Pork fat (lard)

▲ Stick margarine

▲ Shortening

Foods high in solid fats include

▲ Many cheeses

▲ Cream

▲ Ice cream

▲ Well-marbled cuts of meats

▲ Regular ground beef

▲ Bacon

▲ Sausages

▲ Poultry skin

▲ Many baked goods (such as cookies, crackers, doughnuts, pastries, and croissants)

Even though many solid-fat foods supply nutrients, most are high in *saturated fats* and/or *trans fats* and have fewer monounsaturated or polyunsaturated fats. Animal products containing solid fats also contain cholesterol. Foods containing partially hydrogenated vegetable oils usually contain trans fats. (Trans fats can be found in many cakes, cookies, crackers, icings, margarines, and microwave popcorns.) Solid fats tend to raise "bad" (LDL) cholesterol levels in the blood, which in turn increases the risk for heart disease. To lower the risk for heart disease, cut back on foods containing saturated fats, trans fats, and cholesterol.

Counting Solid Fats

The chart on pages 134–135 serves as a quick guide to the amount of solid fats in some common foods. All calories from solid fats count as discretionary calories.

Discretionary Calories from Added Sugars

Added sugars include sugars, syrups, and high-calorie sweeteners that are added to foods or beverages during processing or preparation. They do not include naturally occurring sugars such as those in milk and fruits.

Foods that contain most of the added sugars in American diets are

▲ Regular soft drinks
▲ Candy
▲ Cakes
▲ Cookies
▲ Pies

Counting Solid Fats

Amount of Food		Amount of Solid Fat (tsp./g)	Calories from Solid fat (approximate)	Total Calories (approximate)
Solid fats				
Shortening	1 Tbsp.	3 tsp./13 g	115	115
Butter	1 Tbsp.	2½ tsp./12 g	100	100
Margarine (hard or stick)	1 Tbsp.	2½ tsp./11 g	100	100
Coconut or palm kernel oil	1 Tbsp.	3 tsp./14 g	120	120
Food rich in solid fats				
Heavy cream	1 Tbsp.	1 tsp./5 g	50	50
Half-and-half cream	1 Tbsp.	½ tsp./2 g	15	20
Sour cream	1 Tbsp.	½ tsp./2 g	20	25
Whole milk	1 cup	2 tsp./8 g	70	145
Cheddar cheese	1½ oz.	3 tsp./14 g	125	170

Counting Solid Fats (continued)

	Amount of Food	Amount of Solid Fat (tsp./g)	Calories from Solid fat (approximate)	Total Calories (approximate)
Ice cream, chocolate	1 cup	3 tsp./14 g	125	285
Bacon, cooked	2 slices	1½ tsp./6 g	55	85
Pork sausage	2 links (2 oz.)	3 tsp./14 g	120	165
Hamburger—regular (80% lean)	3 oz., cooked	3 tsp./14 g	120	205
Prime rib roast, lean and fat (⅛" trim)	3 oz., cooked	6 tsp./29 g	255	340
Prime rib roast, lean only	3 oz., cooked	3½ tsp./16 g	140	250
Croissant	1 medium (2 oz.)	3 tsp./12 g	105	230
Biscuit	1 small (2.5" diameter)	1½ tsp./6 g	50	125
Pound cake	½ of 12-oz. cake	1½ tsp./6 g	50	110
Cheese Danish	1 pastry (2½ oz.)	3½ tsp./16 g	135	265
Chocolate cream pie	⅛ of 8" pie	5 tsp./22 g	195	345

▲ Fruit drinks, such as fruitades and fruit punch

▲ Milk-based desserts and products, such as ice cream, sweetened yogurt, and sweetened milk

▲ Grain products such as sweet rolls and cinnamon toast

Reading the ingredients labels on processed foods can help to identify added sugars. Names for added sugars on food labels include

▲ Brown sugar

▲ Corn sweetener

▲ Corn syrup

▲ Dextrose

▲ Fructose

▲ Fruit juice concentrates

▲ Glucose

▲ High-fructose corn syrup

▲ Honey

▲ Invert sugar

▲ Lactose

▲ Maltose

▲ Malt syrup

▲ Molasses

▲ Raw sugar

▲ Sucrose

▲ Sugar

▲ Syrup

Like solid fats, added sugars ladle on calories. Although sugars, being carbohydrates, do supply readily available energy, their nutrient value is usually low.

Discretionary Calories from Alcohol

Alcohol is high in calories and low in nutrients.

Alcohol	Ounces	Calories
Beer	12	146
Gin (90 proof)	1.5	110
Whiskey (86 proof)	1.5	105
Rum (80 proof)	1.5	97
Vodka (80 proof)	1.5	97
Wine, red	4	85
Wine, white	4	80
Champagne	4	79
Cordials (liqueurs)	1.5	146–186

Cocktails and mixed drinks can be even higher in calories because they often contain sweet and creamy additions. Save calories by choosing lower-calorie, lower-fat mixers such as club soda, sparkling water, or orange, lime, lemon, cranberry, vegetable, or tomato juice.

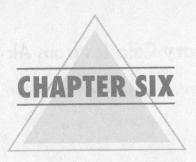

CHAPTER SIX

Earn More Calories and Better Health with Physical Activity

My Pyramid Directive: Get at least thirty minutes of moderate-to-vigorous physical activity every day. Exercise optimizes your health, stamina, longevity, performance, and mental well-being . . . and allows you to eat more.

What Counts as Physical Activity?

Most people know that physical activity and nutrition work together for better health. Yet the old Food Pyramid was only about food and made no provisions for burning calories. Meanwhile, Americans have become more and more sedentary, spending almost their entire lives sitting, either at work, in the car, or slumped on the couch.

The new My Pyramid gets smart. It recommends at least thirty minutes of moderate-to-vigorous physical activity daily. In this case, physical activity means movement of the body that uses energy and increases your heart rate. So, want to eat more cake and french fries? And wash them down with soda and beer? You can "earn" more discretionary calories by getting up and getting some exercise.

Whereas all activity helps reduce health risks and burns calories, My Pyramid calorie and intake recommendations are based on activity that increases your heart rate. In addition, My Pyramid recommends that you do at least ten-minute bouts of the activity at a time. Again, only heart-rate-changing activities count toward the thirty or more minutes a day of moderate-to-vigorous physical activity that My Pyramid suggests.

Moderate physical activities include

▲ Walking briskly (about 3½ miles per hour)

▲ Hiking

▲ Gardening/yard work

▲ Dancing

▲ Golf (walking and carrying clubs)

▲ Bicycling (less than 10 miles per hour)

▲ Weight training (general light workout)

Vigorous physical activities include

▲ Running/jogging (5 miles per hour)

▲ Bicycling (more than 10 miles per hour)

▲ Swimming (freestyle laps)

▲ Aerobics

▲ Walking very fast (4½ miles per hour)

▲ Heavy yard work, such as chopping wood

▲ Weight lifting (vigorous effort)

▲ Basketball (competitive)

Why Is Physical Activity Important?

Physical activity is crucial because our species did not evolve to stay healthy while idle. Only in the last century have humans become sedentary. The evolutionary processes that led to the way we digest and use food took place during times of intense physical activity—hunting, gathering, fighting, fleeing, and traveling. That means we are physically designed for activity that is more strenuous than that in which most people participate. The benefits of physical activity may include

▲ Increasing fitness level

▲ Helping to build and maintain bones, muscles, and joints

▲ Building endurance and muscle strength

▲ Enhancing flexibility and posture

▲ Managing weight

▲ Lowering risk of heart disease, colon cancer, and type 2 diabetes

▲ Helping to control blood pressure

▲ Reducing feelings of depression and anxiety

▲ Relieving stress

▲ Improving self-esteem and feelings of well-being

Different types of physical activity treat different aspects of our well-being:

▲ *Aerobic activities* speed heart rate and breathing, even as they improve heart and lung fitness. Examples are brisk walking, jogging, and swimming.

▲ *Resistance, strength-building, and weight-bearing activities* help build and maintain bones and muscles by strengthening them against the force of gravity. Examples are carrying a child, lifting weights, and walking.

▲ *Balance and stretching activities* enhance physical stability and flexibility, which reduces the risk of injuries. Examples are gentle stretching, dancing, yoga, martial arts, and t'ai chi.

How Does Physical Activity Affect Cholesterol?

Regular physical activity increases HDL cholesterol in some people. (See "Cholesterol" box in the Oils Group section in Chapter 4.) Increased glycogen breakdown in the liver leads to the production of HDL, which is then released into the bloodstream. Physical inactivity is a major risk factor for heart disease. Even moderate-intensity activities, if done daily, help reduce your risk.

Exercise Raises Your Calorie Allotment

In addition to garnering the physical benefits of exercise, people who engage in thirty or more minutes of exercise each day can eat more. The best way to earn more calories is to burn more. As the following chart makes apparent, exercise means you can eat as much as 25 percent more, depending on your age, gender, and activity level.

Calorie Allocation by Age

My Pyramid assigns individuals to a calorie level based on their sex, age, and activity level.

This chart identifies the calorie levels for males and females by age and activity level. Calorie levels are provided for each year of childhood, from two to eighteen years, and for adults in five-year increments.

	Males			Activity Level	Females		
Age	Sedentary*	Moderately active*	Active*	Age	Sedentary*	Moderately active*	Active*
2	1,000	1,000	1,000	2	1,000	1,000	1,000
3	1,000	1,400	1,400	3	1,000	1,200	1,400
4	1,200	1,400	1,600	4	1,200	1,400	1,400
5	1,200	1,400	1,600	5	1,200	1,400	1,600
6	1,400	1,600	1,800	6	1,200	1,400	1,600
7	1,400	1,600	1,800	7	1,200	1,600	1,800
8	1,400	1,600	2,000	8	1,400	1,600	1,800
9	1,600	1,800	2,000	9	1,400	1,600	1,800
10	1,600	1,800	2,200	10	1,400	1,800	2,000
11	1,800	2,000	2,200	11	1,600	1,800	2,000
12	1,800	2,200	2,400	12	1,600	2,000	2,200
13	2,000	2,200	2,600	13	1,600	2,000	2,200
14	2,000	2,400	2,800	14	1,800	2,000	2,400
15	2,200	2,600	3,000	15	1,800	2,000	2,400
16	2,400	2,800	3,200	16	1,800	2,000	2,400
17	2,400	2,800	3,200	17	1,800	2,000	2,400

Calorie Allocation by Age (continued)

Activity Level Age	Males			Activity Level Age	Females		
	Sedentary*	Moderately active*	Active*		Sedentary*	Moderately active*	Active*
18	2,400	2,800	3,200	18	1,800	2,000	2,400
19–20	2,600	2,800	3,000	19–20	2,000	2,200	2,400
21–25	2,400	2,800	3,000	21–25	2,000	2,200	2,400
26–30	2,400	2,600	3,000	26–30	1,800	2,000	2,400
31–35	2,400	2,600	3,000	31–35	1,800	2,000	2,200
36–40	2,400	2,600	2,800	36–40	1,800	2,000	2,200
41–45	2,200	2,600	2,800	41–45	1,800	2,000	2,200
46–50	2,200	2,400	2,800	46–50	1,800	2,000	2,200
51–55	2,200	2,400	2,800	51–55	1,600	1,800	2,200
56–60	2,200	2,400	2,600	56–60	1,600	1,800	2,200
61–65	2,000	2,400	2,600	61–65	1,600	1,800	2,000
66–70	2,000	2,200	2,600	66–70	1,600	1,800	2,000
71–75	2,000	2,200	2,600	71–75	1,600	1,800	2,000
76 and up	2,000	2,200	2,400	76 and up	1,600	1,800	2,000

*Calorie levels are based on the Estimated Energy Requirements (EER) and activity levels from the Institute of Medicine Dietary Reference Intakes Macronutrients Report, 2002.

Sedentary = less than thirty minutes a day of moderate physical activity in addition to daily activities.

Moderately active = at least thirty minutes up to sixty minutes a day of moderate physical activity in addition to daily activities.

Active = Sixty or more minutes a day of moderate physical activity in addition to daily activities.

My Pyramid Food Intake Pattern Calorie Levels

Sedentary means you have a lifestyle that includes only the light physical activity associated with typical day-to-day life.

Moderately active means you have a lifestyle that includes activity but at only slightly faster than normal pace, one that raises the heart rate.

Active means a lifestyle that includes physical activity equivalent to walking more than 3 miles per day at 3 to 4 miles per hour, in addition to the light physical activity associated with typical endeavor.

How Much Physical Activity Is Needed?

Let us assume that you want to achieve your ideal weight, that you also want to be healthy, that you want to live a long life . . . and even that you want to eat more than the Spartan quantities put forward by My Pyramid. If all this is true, then you must shake off any aversion to physical activity and throw away all those excuses you have for not getting any exercise.

If you are already lucky enough to be healthy and at your ideal weight, you still need to exercise to ward off the kinds of problems that develop as a result of our increasingly stressful lifestyles and exposure to pollutants. At a minimum, do *moderate*-intensity activity for thirty minutes every day, or almost every day. Do this in addition to your usual daily activities. Remember, *moderate* doesn't mean walking from the curb to your cubicle; it means raising your heart rate.

By increasing the intensity or the amount of time you exercise, you increase the health benefits. Although thirty minutes a day of moderate-intensity physical activities deliver the advantages, being active for longer and doing more vigorous activities do it even better. They also use up more calories per hour.

More exercise may be required to combat weight gain. Depending on how much you eat, about sixty minutes a day of moderate physical activity may be *your* minimum. For those who have lost weight, maintaining the weight loss may demand at least sixty to ninety minutes of exercise a day. Don't forget that you must always balance calories spent with calories consumed. Do not eat beyond your calorie needs; otherwise, that fitness-center membership will be for nothing.

Children and teenagers should be physically active for at least sixty minutes every day, or most days. And do not think

Cautionary Note

My Pyramid recommends that men over the age of forty and women over the age of fifty should consult a health care provider before commencing a program of vigorous physical activity. Also consult a health care provider for help in designing a safe program of physical activity, if you have either of the following conditions:

▲ *A chronic health problem such as heart disease, high blood pressure, diabetes, osteoporosis, asthma, or obesity*

▲ *A high risk for heart disease, including having a family history of heart disease or stroke; eating a diet high in saturated fat, trans fat, and cholesterol; smoking; or having a sedentary lifestyle.*

you are off the hook when you pass middle age. As people age, their metabolism slows, so maintaining energy balance still requires moving more and eating less, even for the elderly.

No matter which activity you choose, it can be done all at once or divided into two or three sessions during the day. Even ten-minute bouts of activity count toward your total.

How Many Calories Does Physical Activity Use?

A 154-pound man (5'10") will use up about the number of calories listed doing each activity in the following chart. *Those who weigh more will use more calories, and those who weigh less will use fewer.* The calorie values listed include both calories used by the activity and calories used for normal body functioning.

Approximate Calories Used by a 154-Pound Man		
Moderate Physical Activities	**In 1 hour**	**In 30 minutes**
Hiking	370	185
Light gardening/yard work	330	165
Dancing	330	165
Golf (walking and carrying clubs)	330	165
Bicycling (less than 10 mph)	290	145
Walking (3½ mph)	280	140
Weight training (general light workout)	220	110
Stretching	180	90
Running/jogging (5 mph)	590	295
Bicycling (more than 10 mph)	590	295
Swimming (slow freestyle laps)	510	255
Aerobics	480	240
Walking (4½ mph)	460	230
Heavy yard work (chopping wood)	440	220
Weight lifting (vigorous effort)	440	220
Basketball (vigorous)	440	220

Treat Stress with Activity

Stress, weight gain, and disease are closely related. Here is why: Over millions of years, humans evolved a "fight or flight" response to stress. The humans who were the most efficient at responding to, for example, a fire or a saber-toothed tiger attack lived and had children. Of their children, those who were best-adapted to stress lived long enough to have children, and so forth. Our ancestors survived because their heart rates went up, their cholesterol rose, and their systems flooded with hormones, all equipping them to accomplish immediate strenuous tasks. Now, all these years later, the saber-toothed tigers are gone, but we still experience stress. Traffic, workaday anxiety, money troubles, and so on, all trigger the same physiological changes. The problem is that we no longer employ these changes in physical endeavors. Instead, we just sit and fret while the changes lead to weight gain and disease. The best thing you can do with your stress is to take action—physical action. Do not eat. Run, skip, jump, or dance. Do anything to make use of the internal stress response.

Tips for Increasing Physical Activity

Make daily physical activity a routine by . . .

▲ Choosing activities that you enjoy and can do regularly.

▲ Exercising with people whose company you enjoy or by yourself, if you prefer.

▲ Keeping it interesting by engaging in a variety of activities and trying something different on alternate days. For example, to reach a thirty-minute goal for the day, walk the dog for ten minutes before and after work, and add a ten-minute walk at lunchtime. Or swim three times a week and take a yoga class on the other days.

▲ Being ready anytime by keeping some comfortable clothes and a pair of walking or running shoes in the car and at the office. You may feel like a ten-minute run at lunchtime or decide to work off some stress in the stairwell during a break.

Ideas for Incorporating More Activity into Busy Schedules

At home:

▲ Join a walking group in the neighborhood or at the local shopping mall.

▲ Recruit a partner for support and encouragement.

▲ Push the baby in a stroller.

▲ Get the whole family involved—enjoy an afternoon bike ride with your kids.

▲ Walk up and down the soccer or softball field sidelines while watching the kids play.

▲ Walk the dog; don't just watch the dog walk.

▲ Clean the house or wash the car, but set a time limit to encourage you to work vigorously.

▲ Walk, skate, or cycle more, and drive less.

▲ Do stretches, exercises, or pedal a stationary bike while watching television.

▲ Mow the lawn with a push mower.

▲ Plant and care for a vegetable or flower garden.

▲ Get involved in community service projects—cleanups and plantings expend calories.

▲ Play with the kids—tumble in the leaves, build a snowman, splash in a puddle, or dance to favorite music.

At work:

▲ Get off the bus or subway one stop early and walk or skate the rest of the way.

▲ Take a brisk ten-minute walk to and from the parking lot, bus stop, or subway station.

▲ Replace a coffee break with a brisk ten-minute walk. Ask a friend to go with you.

▲ Take part in an exercise program at work or a nearby gym.

▲ Join the office softball or bowling team.

▲ Use a fitness ball as a chair.

At play:

▲ Walk, jog, skate, or cycle.

▲ Swim or do water aerobics.

▲ Attend regularly scheduled classes in martial arts, dance, yoga, tap, kickboxing, basketball, or the like.

▲ Golf (pull a cart or carry your clubs).

▲ Canoe, row, or kayak.

▲ Play racquetball, tennis, or squash.

▲ Ski cross-country or downhill.

▲ Play basketball, softball, or soccer.

▲ Hand cycle or play wheelchair sports.

▲ Take a nature walk.

Most important, congratulate yourself for doing something so good for yourself. Knowing that the time you spend exercising is contributing to better looks and a better future should make it fun to be active!

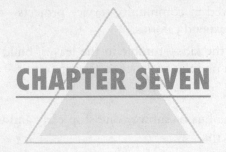

CHAPTER SEVEN

Understanding the Nutrition Facts Label

You think it's hard to make sure your family eats well? Imagine having the nutritional welfare of nearly three hundred million people as a responsibility, as does the U.S. Food and Drug Administration (FDA) Center for Food Safety and Applied Nutrition. The Nutrition Facts label on food bags, cans, jars, and bottles is the FDA's best effort to keep Americans' nutrition on track.

Manufacturers used to be able to plaster all kinds of claims on food packaging, but since the passage of the Nutrition Labeling and Education Act in 1990, the FDA must *approve* those claims. The act also standardized nutrition labels. Manufacturers can no longer camouflage substances in a jungle of multiletter ingredients. In the years since this standardization, manufacturers have been offering more nutritional foods; however, the number of packaged and processed foods has likewise increased. Obviously, food labels do not do all our thinking for us. We still have to think (and eat!) between the lines.

If you want to know whether the product is good for you, look at the label.

The FDA has done its best to make sure food product labels have something for everyone. The results are fairly comprehensive, but can be somewhat of a head-scratcher.

To learn how to use food-label information more effectively and easily, consumers need label-reading skills. The following explanations, distilled from FDA guidelines, will make it easier for you to make quick, informed food choices that contribute to a healthy diet.

Overview of a Nutrition Facts Label

Before investigating each section separately, let's analyze the anatomy of the label, based on the following sample nutrition label for macaroni and cheese.

The main, or top, section (see circled numbers 1 through 4 and 6 on the sample nutrition label, on the next page) contains product-specific information (serving size, calories, and nutrient information) and varies with each food product. The bottom part (see circled number 5 on the sample label) contains a footnote with Daily Values (DVs). The footnote is found only on larger packages and does not change from product to product. This footnote lets you know the upper limits for fats, cholesterol, and sodium, as well as how much fiber is recommended, for 2,000- and 2,500-calorie diets. Caution: These caloric recommendations apply to moderately active adult men and women. Before puberty, children will need less; inactive adults also require less.

Here is an introduction to the Nutrition Facts elements and the Percent Daily Value (% DV).

Sample label for
Macaroni & Cheese

Nutrition Facts

1. Start
   Here

Serving Size 1 cup (228g)
Servings Per Container 2

2. Check
   Calories

Amount Per Serving

Calories 250   Calories from Fat 110

	% Daily Value*
Total Fat 12g	18%
Saturated Fat 3g	15%
Trans Fat 3g	
Cholesterol 30mg	10%
Sodium 470mg	20%
Total Carbohydrate 31g	10%

3. Limit
   These
   Nutrients

6. Quick
   Guide to
   % DV

▲ 5% or
   Less Is
   Low

▲ 20% or
   More Is
   High

Dietary Fiber 0g	0%
Sugars 5g	
Protein 5g	
Vitamin A	4%
Vitamin C	2%
Calcium	20%
Iron	4%

4. Get
   Enough of
   These
   Nutrients

5. Footnote

*Percent Daily Values are based on a 2,000 calorie diet.
Your Daily Values may be higher or lower depending on
your calorie needs.

	Calories:	2,000	2,500
Total Fat	Less than	65g	80g
Sat Fat	Less than	20g	25g
Cholesterol	Less than	300mg	300mg
Sodium	Less than	2,400mg	2,400mg
Total Carbohydrate		300g	375g
Dietary Fiber		25g	30g

Nutrition Facts
Serving Size 1 cup (228g)
Servings Per Container 2

❶ How Big Is the Serving Size and How Many Servings Per Container?

Start at the top by looking at the *serving size* and the *number of servings* in the package. Standardized serving sizes make it easier to compare similar foods; they are provided in familiar units, such as cups or pieces, followed by the metric amount, for example, the number of grams.

It may be that the serving size listed on the package is smaller than the amount you are actually eating. If you neglect to correlate your serving size with the amount on the label, you

	Example			
	Single Serving	*% DV*	*Double Serving*	*% DV*
Serving size	1 cup (228 g)		2 cups (456 g)	
Calories	250		500	
Calories from fat	110		220	
Total fat	12 g	18%	24 g	36%
Trans fat	1.5 g		3 g	
Saturated fat	3 g	15%	6 g	30%
Cholesterol	30 mg	10%	60 mg	20%
Sodium	470 mg	20%	940 mg	40%
Total carbohydrate	31 g	10%	62 g	20%
Dietary fiber	0 g	0%	0 g	0%
Sugars	5 g		10 g	
Protein	5 g		10 g	
Vitamin A		4%		8%
Vitamin C		2%		4%
Calcium		20%		40%
Iron		4%		8%

will sabotage your work to keep within My Pyramid calorie limits. *Pay attention to the specified serving size, especially to how many servings there are in the food package. Then ask yourself, "How many servings am I consuming?" (e.g., ½ serving, 1 serving, or more).*

The size of the serving indicated on the food package determines the number of calories and all the nutrient amounts listed on the top part of the label. On the sample label, one serving of macaroni and cheese equals 1 cup. If you ate the whole package, you would eat 2 cups. That doubles the calories and other nutrient numbers, including the Percent Daily Values as shown on the sample label. The label is not going to do arithmetic for you; if you do not eat the specified serving size, you will have to do some math.

❷ *How Many* Calories *and* Calories from Fat

Calories provide a measure of how much energy you get from a serving of this food. *Eating too many calories per day is linked to being overweight or obese.* The calorie section of the label can help you manage your weight (i.e., gain, lose, or maintain it). Many Americans consume more calories than they need without meeting recommended intakes for a number of nutrients, as you know from previous chapters. By specifying the number of *calories from fat,* the label is trying to help you eat healthier. Ideally, your calories-from-fat intake should be only 30 percent of your total caloric intake. *Remember: The number of servings you consume determines the number of calories you actually eat (your portion amount).*

Continuing the macaroni and cheese example, there are 250 calories in one serving of this macaroni and cheese. Of these, 110 calories are from fat. Almost half the calories in a single serving come from fat—50 percent. To decrease the 50 percent to 30 percent, the other foods you eat with the macaroni and cheese and the rest of the day must have significantly fewer calories from fat. If you ate the whole package content, you would consume two servings, or 500 calories, and 220 of them would come from fat.

General Guide to Calories

▲ *40 calories is low.*

▲ *100 calories is moderate.*

▲ *400 calories or more is high.*

The General Guide to Calories provides a general reference for calories when you look at a Nutrition Facts label. This guide is based on a 2,000-calorie diet.

How Many Nutrients?

The *nutrient* section on the sample label shows you some key nutrients that impact your health. It separates these into two main groups: those we should eat in moderation and those we should strive to eat more abundantly. *You can use the Nutrition Facts label to help* limit *those nutrients you want to cut back on and also to* increase *those nutrients you need to consume in greater amounts.*

❸ First on the list are those nutrients Americans usually eat in sufficient quantities or even eat too much of. These are here because they are problematic. Eating too much fat, saturated fat, trans fat, cholesterol, or sodium may increase your risk of certain chronic diseases, such as heart disease, some cancers, or high blood pressure. The label does not say eating foods high in these nutrients is hazardous to your health, but it can be.

	% Daily Value*
Total Fat 12g	18%
Saturated Fat 3g	15%
Trans Fat 3g	
Cholesterol 30mg	10%
Sodium 470mg	20%
Total Carbohydrate 31g	10%

Important: Health experts recommend that you keep your intake of saturated fat, trans fat, and cholesterol as low as possible as part of a nutritionally balanced diet. Some product labels include line items for polyunsaturated and monounsaturated fats. Unlike saturated fats and trans fats, these fats are actually good for us, as you know from Chapter 4. They are, however, still high in calories and should be consumed only in moderation.

Reading labels is particularly important for people who must limit salt intake (to control hypertension), because most sodium (salt) in the food supply comes from packaged foods. Similar packaged foods, such as breads, can vary widely in sodium content. A claim such as "low in sodium" or "very low in sodium" on the front of the food label can help you identify foods that contain less salt (or sodium). Foods with less than 140 milligrams of sodium per serving can be labeled as low-sodium foods.

The *% Daily Value* on the right side of the label tells how much of the recommended daily amount of the nutrient is in one serving, based on a 2,000-calorie diet. If you follow this dietary advice, you will stay within public health experts' recommended upper or lower limits for the nutrients listed, as long as you are eating a 2,000-calorie daily diet. If you are *not* eating a 2,000-calorie diet, you will need to adjust these up or down. Here is the formula for figuring out what percentage of your Daily Value one serving supplies:

$$\frac{2,000}{\text{Your Total Daily Calories}} \times \text{Amount in Daily Value Column}$$
$$= \text{Percentage of Your Daily Value}$$
$$\text{Supplied by One Serving}$$
$$\text{of the Food}$$

For example, the macaroni and cheese label indicates that one serving supplies 10 percent of the Daily Value (Recommended Daily Allowance) of cholesterol. Let's say you eat 1,600 calories instead of 2,000. Divide 2,000 by 1,600 and get 1.25. Multiply 10 by 1.25 and get 12.5. This means one serving of macaroni supplies 12.5 percent of the Daily Value, or Recommended Daily Allowance, for a 1,600-calorie diet.

If, instead, small portions are your objective, here is the formula for reducing the serving size, to keep the Percent Daily Value consistent:

$$\frac{\text{Your Total Calories Daily}}{2,000} \times \text{Serving Size on Package}$$
$$= \text{Your Reduced Serving Size}$$

The macaroni and cheese label indicates that one serving is 228 grams, or 1 cup. Again, let's say you eat 1,600 calories instead of 2,000. Divide 1,600 by 2,000 and get 0.8. Multiply 1 cup by 0.8 and get ⅘ cup, or 182.4 grams. This means one ⅘-cup serving of macaroni will still supply 10 percent of your Daily Value, or Recommended Daily Allowance, for a 1,600-calorie diet.

The asterisk (*) refers to the footnote on the lower part of the nutrition label, which tells you the recommended DVs based on a 2,000-calorie diet and a 2,500-calorie diet only. This footnote may not be on the package if the label is too small.

❹ You probably eat all the sugar and protein you need. Note that most labels have no % DV for sugar and protein. Some have % DV for protein if the product makes and meets protein-content claims. However, among the second bank of nutrients are some that people should eat more abundantly.

Dietary Fiber 0g	0%
Sugars 5g	
Protein 5g	
Vitamin A	4%
Vitamin C	2%
Calcium	20%
Iron	4%

Most Americans do not get enough dietary fiber, vitamin A, vitamin C, calcium, or iron in their diets. Eating enough of these nutrients can improve your health and help reduce the risk of some diseases and conditions. For example, a diet rich in fruits, vegetables, and grain products that contain dietary fiber, particularly soluble fiber, and are low in saturated fat and cholesterol may reduce the risk of heart disease. Eating a diet high in fiber promotes healthy bowel function. Additionally, getting enough calcium may reduce the risk of osteoporosis, a condition that results in brittle bones as one ages. The % DV on food packages makes it easy to recognize how much one serving contributes to the total amount of these nutrients that you need per day.

Do not make assumptions about the amount of nutrients in specific food categories. For example, the amount of calcium in milk, whether skim or whole, is generally the same per serving, whereas the amount of calcium in the same size yogurt container (8 ounces) can vary from 20 to 45% DV. Check the labels!

❺ *Understanding the Daily Value Footnote*

Many, but not all, packages have a footnote on the lower part of the label telling how much fat, saturated fat, cholesterol, sodium, carbohydrate, and fiber should be included in 2,000-calorie and 2,500-calorie daily diets. The footnote may not be on the package if the label is too small. However, the information in the footnote is always the same and never varies from label to label. It shows recommended dietary advice for all Americans—it is not about a specific food product.

The footnote is provided to help you relate the percentages asterisks (*), which are to the right of the nutrients in the upper part of the label, to Daily Values. Daily Values are actually Recommended Daily Allowances, in grams and milligrams.

*Percent Daily Values are based on a 2,000 calorie diet. Your Daily Values may be higher or lower depending on your calorie needs.			
	Calories:	2,000	2,500
Total Fat	Less than	65g	80g
Sat Fat	Less than	20g	25g
Cholesterol	Less than	300mg	300mg
Sodium	Less than	2,400mg	2,400mg
Total Carbohydrate		300g	375g
Dietary Fiber		25g	30g

Note how the DVs for some nutrients change, while others (for cholesterol and sodium) remain the same for both calorie amounts.

If you follow this dietary advice, you will stay within public health experts' recommended upper or lower limits for the nutrients listed, based on a 2,000-calorie daily diet.

Eat "Less Than"

The nutrients that have upper daily limits are listed first on the footnote. Upper limits mean that it is recommended that you stay below, or eat less than, the Daily Value nutrient amounts listed per day. For example, the DV for saturated fat ("Sat Fat") is 20 grams for a 2,000-calorie diet. This amount is 100% DV for this nutrient. The goal is to eat less than 20 grams, or 100% DV, for the day.

Eat "At Least"

My Pyramid recommends that we eat more complex carbohydrates and more fiber. Therefore, it does not have a "less than" limitation on carbs and fiber on the label. The DV for carbohydrate is 300 grams, which is 100% DV for a 2,000-calorie diet. The DV for dietary fiber is 25 grams, which is 100% DV for a 2,000-calorie diet. This means it is recommended that you eat at least this amount of dietary fiber per day.

The DV for total carbohydrate (section in white) is 300 grams, or 100% DV. This amount is recommended for a balanced daily diet that is based on 2,000 calories, but it can vary, depending on your daily intake of fat and protein.

As you begin paying attention to % DVs, you will notice how often you get too much of those nutrients you want to limit (e.g., fat, saturated fat, cholesterol, and sodium). Likewise, you will probably note that you do not necessarily get enough of those that you want to consume in greater amounts (fiber, calcium, etc.). On any product label, 5% DV or less is low and 20% or more is high for all nutrients.

For example, look at the amount of total fat in one serving listed on the sample nutrition label. A DV of 18%, which is below 20% DV, is not yet high, but what if you ate the whole

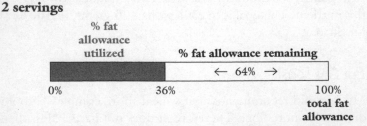

package (two servings)? You would double that amount, eating 36 percent of your daily allowance for total fat. Coming from just one food, that amount leaves you with 64 percent of your fat allowance (100% − 36% = 64%) for *all* of the other foods you eat that day, snacks and drinks included.

In creating the Percent Daily Value, the Food and Drug Administration standardized labels to help consumers do the following:

1. *Verify nutrient content:* Instead of having to memorize definitions, you can use the % DV to distinguish one claim from another, such as "reduced fat" versus "light" or "nonfat." Just compare the % DVs for total fat in each food product to see which one is higher or lower in that nutrient.

2. *Satisfy daily dietary requirements:* You can use the % DV to help you make dietary trade-offs with other foods throughout the day. You don't have to give up a favorite food to eat a healthy diet. When a food you like is high in fat, balance it with foods that are low in fat at other times of the day. Pay attention to how much you eat so that the *total* amount of fat for the day stays below 100% DV.

3. *Compare products:* The % DV can guide you in comparisons between one product or brand and similar products. Make sure the serving sizes are similar, especially the weight (e.g., grams, milligrams, ounces) of each product. It is easy to see which foods are higher or lower in nutrients because the serving sizes are generally consistent for similar types of foods (see the comparison example at the end of this chapter), except in a few cases like cereals.

For example, the following labels are for two kinds of milk—one is reduced-fat and the other is chocolate nonfat milk. Each serving size is 1 cup. Note that while their calcium content is the same, their calories and saturated fat are different.

REDUCED-FAT MILK

2% MILKFAT   CHOCOLATE NONFAT MILK

Nutrition Facts	
Serving Size 1 cup (236ml)	
Servings Per Container 1	
Amount Per Serving	
Calories 120	Calories from Fat 45
	% Daily Value*
Total Fat 5g	**8%**
Saturated Fat 3g	**15%**
Trans Fat 0g	
Cholesterol 20mg	7%
Sodium 120mg	5%
Total Carbohydrate 11g	4%
Dietary Fiber 0g	0%
Sugars 11g	
Protein 9g	17%
Vitamin A 10% • Vitamin C 4%	
Calcium 30% • Iron 0% • Vitamin D 25%	
*Percent Daily Values are based on a 2,000 calorie diet. Your Daily Values may be higher or lower depending on your calorie needs.	

Nutrition Facts	
Serving Size 1 cup (236ml)	
Servings Per Container 1	
Amount Per Serving	
Calories 80	Calories from Fat 0
	% Daily Value*
Total Fat 0g	**0%**
Saturated Fat 0g	**0%**
Trans Fat 0g	
Cholesterol Less than 5mg	0%
Sodium 120mg	5%
Total Carbohydrate 11g	4%
Dietary Fiber 0g	0%
Sugars 11g	
Protein 9g	17%
Vitamin A 10% • Vitamin C 4%	
Calcium 30% • Iron 0% • Vitamin D 25%	
*Percent Daily Values are based on a 2,000 calorie diet. Your Daily Values may be higher or lower depending on your calorie needs.	

Nutrients without a % DV: Note that trans fat, sugars, and protein do not list a % DV on the Nutrition Facts label.

Trans fat: Scientific reports link trans fat (and saturated fat) with raising blood LDL ("bad") cholesterol levels, and both increase your risk of coronary heart disease, a leading cause of death in the United States. Therefore, there is no % DV.

> **Important: Health experts recommend that you keep your intake of saturated fat, trans fat, and cholesterol as low as possible as part of a nutritionally balanced diet.**

Protein: Current scientific evidence indicates that protein intake is not a public health concern for adults and children over four years of age because Americans usually eat more protein than they need.

PLAIN YOGURT

Nutrition Facts
Serving Size 1 container (226g)

Amount Per Serving

Calories 110   Calories from Fat 0

% Daily Value*

Total Fat 0g	0%
Saturated Fat 0g	0%
Trans Fat 0g	
Cholesterol Less than 5mg	1%
Sodium 160mg	7%
Total Carbohydrate 15g	5%
Dietary Fiber 0g	0%
Sugars 10g	
Protein 13g	

Vitamin A	0%	Vitamin C	4%
Calcium	45%	Iron	0%

*Percent Daily Values are based on a 2,000 calorie diet. Your Daily Values may be higher or lower depending on your calorie needs.

FRUIT YOGURT

Nutrition Facts
Serving Size 1 container (227g)

Amount Per Serving

Calories 240   Calories from Fat 25

% Daily Value*

Total Fat 3g	4%
Saturated Fat 1.5g	9%
Trans Fat 0g	
Cholesterol 15mg	5%
Sodium 140mg	6%
Total Carbohydrate 46g	15%
Dietary Fiber Less than 1g	3%
Sugars 44g	
Protein 9g	

Vitamin A	2%	Vitamin C	4%
Calcium	35%	Iron	0%

*Percent Daily Values are based on a 2,000 calorie diet. Your Daily Values may be higher or lower depending on your calorie needs.

Therefore, the % DV is required only if a claim is made for protein, such as "high in protein." Otherwise, unless the food is meant for use by infants and children under four years old, none is needed.

Sugars: No daily reference value has been established for sugars because no recommendations have been made for the total amount to eat in a day.

Sugars are a particular concern to people with diabetes. Keep in mind that the sugars listed on the Nutrition Facts label include naturally occurring sugars (like those in fruit and milk) as well as those added to a food or drink. Check the ingredient list for specifics on added sugars.

Take a look at the Nutrition Facts label for the two yogurt examples. The plain yogurt on the left has 10 grams of sugars, while the fruit yogurt on the right has 44 grams of sugars in one serving.

Now look at the following ingredient lists for the two yogurts. Ingredients are listed in descending order of weight (from most to least). Note that no added sugars or sweeteners are in the list of ingredients for the plain yogurt, yet 10 grams of sugars were listed on the Nutrition Facts label. This is because there are no added sugars in plain yogurt, only naturally occurring sugars (lactose in the milk).

PLAIN YOGURT—CONTAINS NO ADDED SUGARS

INGREDIENTS: CULTURED PASTEURIZED GRADE A NONFAT MILK, WHEY PROTEIN CONCENTRATE, PECTIN, CARRAGEENAN.

FRUIT YOGURT—CONTAINS ADDED SUGARS

INGREDIENTS: CULTURED GRADE A REDUCED FAT MILK, APPLES, HIGH FRUCTOSE CORN SYRUP, CINNAMON, NUTMEG, NATURAL FLAVORS, AND PECTIN. CONTAINS ACTIVE YOGURT AND L. ACIDOPHILUS CULTURES.

If you are concerned about your intake of sugars, make sure that added sugars are not listed as one of the first few ingredients. Other names for added sugars include *corn syrup, high-fructose corn syrup, fruit juice concentrate, maltose, dextrose, sucrose, honey,* and *maple syrup.*

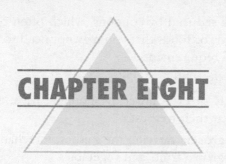

CHAPTER EIGHT

Getting the Most Out of Every Mouthful

My Pyramid makes it clearer than ever that we cannot eat just anything—putting blind trust in agribusiness, grocers, manufacturers, and restaurants—and remain healthy. Yet as complicated as eating well has become, you can still achieve it at home with careful *shopping, storing,* and *preparation.*

Shopping Tips

▲ Plan healthy meals ahead, getting ideas from cookbooks and magazines.

▲ Keep a running list of items you need in your kitchen. Organize the list by category to match your store layout, prioritizing produce and grains.

▲ Do not be seduced by coupons, which often promote processed foods or foods that you may not need to achieve your nutritional requirements.

▲ Take your list with you to the store.

▲ Plan weekly or even biweekly shopping trips, to make sure goods are at their freshest.

▲ Buy from grocers carrying the freshest merchandise:
  ● Locally grown fruits and vegetables
  ● Organically grown fruits and vegetables
  ● Organic meat and poultry and fresh fish
  ● Unprocessed food
    This should be easy since one-third of the two million farms in the United States are located within metropolitan areas and produce 35 percent of U.S. vegetables, fruit, livestock, poultry, and fish.[30]

▲ Make frozen goods, not canned goods (which have more sodium), your second choice after fresh goods.

▲ Choose low-fat or nonfat dairy products.

▲ Purchase legumes and soy products to prepare meatless dishes.

▲ Buy seafood with firm flesh and a fresh smell.

▲ Buy lean meats only.

▲ Do not buy meat by its color. Meat should smell fresh and not be slimy. Read labels and avoid meats with injected water, flavorings, and preservatives. Local butcher shops—particularly those that carry organic meats or meat from grass-fed or free-range animals—may be the best option.

▲ Poultry is often a good choice, but remember that grocery store poultry usually has a lot of fat. Buy skinless.

▲ Buy whole-grain breads, cereals, and grains. Health-food stores are a good source of bulk grains.

▲ Replenish supplies of unsaturated oils, including olive oil, safflower oil, nut oils, and sesame seed oil.

▲ Assure yourself of savory dishes by keeping a variety of spices, including garlic, onions, shallots, low-sodium tamari, and hot sauce, on hand.

▲ Stay away from the grocery aisles that contain snacks, sodas, and baked goods.

▲ For snacks, purchase vegetables with dips, nuts, and whole-grain crackers.

▲ For drinks, purchase juices and bubbly waters.

▲ For treats, purchase fruits and dried fruits.

▲ Focus on top nutritional value, not discounts.

▲ Keep raw meat, poultry, seafood, and eggs separate from ready-to-eat foods in your grocery shopping cart and your grocery bags. Consider placing these raw foods inside plastic bags to keep the juices contained.

Frozen Food

Freezing retains more nutrient value than other forms of processing. However, frozen vegetables lose from one-third to three-quarters of their vitamin C content if stored for a year.[31] Other nutrient losses occur either in the processing prior to freezing or in the cooking once the frozen food is thawed. Packaged frozen food is characteristically processed almost immediately after harvest and may have more nutrient value than produce that has deteriorated since its harvest. Therefore, if you do not intend to eat very fresh produce or when fresh produce is out of your price range, frozen and even canned goods are good alternatives.

▲ Transport food home right away and refrigerate perishables immediately to preserve freshness and prevent any bacteria from rapidly multiplying in the food. In hot weather, place the groceries in the air-conditioned compartment of your car rather than the hot trunk.

▲ After you get home, have a look at this list again and see whether you shopped successfully.

Seasonal Foods

Eating food seasonally will keep you focused on fresh options. Generally, the warmer the weather, the lighter the fare. Grill during as much of the year as weather allows. Save the heavy soups, stews, casseroles, and stuffed meat dishes for winter.

Spring foods: *Light lamb, white meats such as chicken and turkey breasts; small birds such as Cornish game hens, squab, and doves; scallops; crab; mussels and clams; king salmon; northern halibut; soft-shelled crabs; sea bass; sole; leeks; asparagus; watercress; new potatoes; artichokes; peas; salad greens; and rhubarb, pineapple, strawberries, and raspberries.*

Summer foods: *Lamb, filet steaks, freshwater bass, trout, lobster, filet of sole, scallops, albacore, shrimp, yellowtail, sardines, beets, corn, radishes, tomatoes, basil, cucumbers, peppers, green beans, zucchini, apricots, cherries, berries, peaches, plums, melons, and nectarines.*

Autumn foods: *Ham, duckling, duck, chicken, pheasant, beef and pork tenderloins, rabbit, venison, red snap-*

per, California lobster, mussels, white sea bass, yellowfin tuna, walnuts, pecans, almonds, eggplant, fava beans, squashes, potatoes, mushrooms, pumpkin, figs, apples, and grapes.

Winter foods: Beef and pork roasts, chops, chicken and calf's liver, buffalo, turkey, mackerel, herring, salmon, smelts, oysters, king crab, Dungeness crab, king salmon, clams, chestnuts, potatoes, endive, spinach, fennel, Brussels sprouts, white beans, lima beans, parsnips, carrots, cauliflower, broccoli, celery root, cabbage, turnips, pears, and citrus fruits such as grapefruits and oranges.

Snacks

As long as we allow ourselves unlimited treats, they will deliver the excess fat, sugar, and salt that chew up discretionary calories and put the calorie budget on tilt. It is wiser to use snack time as an opportunity to meet daily requirements for vegetables and fruit. Instead of laying in stores of salty snacks filled with processed ingredients, chocolate, ice cream, cookies, and other baked goods, make sure you buy plenty of veggies and dip, yogurt and fruit, and nuts. Buy small containers to transport them to work and school. Snacking this way, you and your family will have more energy and more stamina . . . and less unwanted weight.

Storage Tips

Consider the real reasons that drive you and your family to reach for chips, baked goods, and sodas. Think about the circumstances under which you resort to ordering pizza or storming the fast-food queues. The fact is that beyond a yearning for rich foods, Americans eat these foods because *they are there,* with no preparation involved.

Thus, one of the biggest steps in your conversion to healthful food is making it easily available and ready to eat. This is where *storage* comes in. Storage has always been about preserving freshness, and certainly those rules still apply (see "Convenience Measures"). However, to accommodate the frantic pace of our modern lives, storage has come to be about convenience, too. Your goal is to have healthful meals and snacks ready (or almost ready). Store them where you and your family will see them.

Convenience Measures

▲ Stock up on stackable, clear (see-through) containers at one of the storage specialty shops, which carry wide arrays of containers and organizers.

▲ When you get home from the market, or the next day, process some veggies and fruits, by cutting them up and storing them.

▲ For snacks, always keep a container of prepared veggies next to hummus or another bean dip, not in the vegetable drawer, but out on a shelf where you and your family will see it.

▲ For snacks and desserts, always keep a container of fruit salad, not in the vegetable drawer but out on a shelf where you and your family will see it.

▲ Have low-fat yogurt and cottage cheese on hand to eat with fruit for a quick breakfast, dessert, or snack.

▲ Store precooked brown rice and other grains, which can be enhanced with other ingredients and reheated for side dishes.

▲ Keep containers of vitamin-rich homemade soups refrigerated and frozen.

▲ Keep nut butters and whole-grain breads on hand for quick sandwiches.

▲ Repackage meat, poultry, and fish into single or family-size portions in freezer wrap. Freeze these portions to use later.

▲ Wrap and freeze whole-grain bread that you cannot use right away.

▲ Among shelf goods, keep whole-grain pasta, quinoa, and bulgur.

▲ Store cereal and grain products in *opaque* containers to avoid exposure to light, which destroys riboflavin and vitamin E.

Freshness Measures

▲ Keep your refrigerator at a temperature of 41°F (5°C) or lower, to slow the growth of bacteria. The freezer should be 0°F (−18°C).

▲ Wrap and seal foods tightly. Always store foods in airtight containers, since oxygen contributes to nutrient depletion. When using plastic bags, push all the air out before sealing.

▲ Always check the labels on cans or jars to determine how the contents should be stored.

▲ Store eggs in their carton in the refrigerator itself rather than on the door, where the temperature is warmer.

▲ Seafood should always be kept in the refrigerator or freezer until preparation time.

▲ Poultry and meat may be stored as purchased in the plastic wrap for a day or two. If only part of the meat or poultry is going to be used right away, it can be wrapped loosely for refrigerator storage. Just make sure juices cannot escape to contaminate other foods.

▲ Many items besides fresh meats, vegetables, and dairy products need to be kept cold. For instance, mayonnaise and ketchup should go in the refrigerator after opening. If you have neglected to refrigerate items, it is usually best to throw them out.

▲ Avoid cross-contamination by keeping raw meat, poultry, and seafood separate from other foods in the refrigerator.

▲ Never taste food that looks or smells strange. Just discard it.

▲ Most moldy food should be discarded. However, you can sometimes save hard cheese, salamis, fruits, and vegetables by cutting the mold out and removing a large area around it.

▲ Do not cram the refrigerator full. Cool air must circulate to keep food safe.

▲ Refrigerate hot foods within two hours after cooking them.

▲ Date leftovers so they can be used within a healthy period of time, usually not more than three days.

▲ Refrigerate or freeze perishables, prepared foods, and leftovers within two hours.

▲ Freezing does not reduce nutrients (except vitamin C). For meat and poultry products, there is little change in protein value during freezing.

▲ Tenderness, flavor, aroma, juiciness, and the color of frozen foods can all be affected by lengthy freezer storage. Freezer burn occurs when air reaches the food's surface and dries out the product. This can happen when food is not securely wrapped in airtight packaging. Color changes result from chemical changes in the food's pigment. Although undesirable, freezer burn does not make the food unsafe. It merely causes dry spots in foods. Cut away these areas either before or after cooking the food.

▲ Never defrost or marinate foods on the counter. Use the refrigerator, cold running water, or a microwave oven.

▲ Divide large amounts of leftovers into small, shallow containers for quick cooling in the refrigerator.

▲ Remove stuffing from poultry and other stuffed meats after cooking and refrigerate in a separate container.

▲ Foods that should be stored at room temperature should not be kept near household cleaning products and chemicals.

▲ Store potatoes and onions in a cool, dry place, not in the refrigerator and not under the sink because leakage from the pipes can damage the food.

▲ Check canned goods to see whether any are sticky on the outside. This may indicate a leak. Newly purchased cans that appear to be leaking should be returned to the store.

▲ Adhere to the "best if used by" date on the label of the product.

Storage Recommendations

| | Storage Period | |
| | In Refrigerator | In Freezer |
Product	40°F (5°C)	0°F (−18°C)
Fresh meat:		
Beef:		
Ground	1–2 days	3–4 months
Steaks and roasts	3–5 days	6–12 months
Pork:		
Chops	3–5 days	4–6 months
Ground	1–2 days	3–4 months
Roasts	3–5 days	4–6 months
Cured meats:		
Lunch meat	3–5 days	1–2 months
Sausage	1–2 days	1–2 months
Gravy	1–2 days	2–3 months

| Product | Storage Period | |
	In Refrigerator 40°F (5°C)	In Freezer 0°F (−18°C)
Fish:		
Lean (such as cod, flounder, haddock)	1–2 days	Up to 6 months 2–3 months
Fatty (such as blue, perch, salmon)	1–2 days	2–3 months
Chicken:		
Whole	1–2 days	12 months
Parts	1–2 days	9 months
Giblets	1–2 days	3–4 months
Dairy products:		
Swiss, brick, processed cheese	3–4 weeks	*
Milk	5 days	1 month
Ice cream, ice milk	—	2–4 months
Eggs:		
Fresh in shell	3 weeks	—
Hard-boiled	1 week	—

*Cheese can be frozen, but freezing will affect the texture and taste.

(*Sources:* Food Marketing Institute for fish and dairy products; USDA for all other foods.)

Preparation Tips

As My Pyramid makes clear, eating healthfully is much more than a matter of a microwave zap and chewing. Careful prepa-

Reheating Reduces Nutrients

Cooked vegetables reheated after two or three days lose up to one-half of their vitamin C and 40 percent of folate.[32]

ration is key in preserving vitamins and enhancing digestibility. Cooking often alters food value, sometimes decreasing and sometimes increasing its healthfulness.

In addition to making food tastier, conscientious cooking . . .

▲ Destroys bacteria and other potentially harmful microorganisms

▲ Breaks down parts of vegetables and grains that would otherwise be indigestible, loosening chemical bonds and releasing more nutrients

▲ Makes beta-carotene, lycopene, iron, calcium, and magnesium more absorbable

▲ Raises the bioavailability of carbohydrates in starches, making their fuel more easily utilized

It is vegetables and fruits that require such care to remain nutrient-rich. In produce, the bulk of the nutrients (vitamins and minerals) is in the outer leaves and close to the skin surface. Overzealous trimming and peeling greatly reduces a vegetable's or a fruit's nutrient value.

Boiling is the number one source of nutrient loss in fruits and vegetables because some vitamins dissolve readily in water. Boiling vegetables boils away the nutrients. Grilling, roasting, steaming, stir-frying, and microwaving generally preserve a greater amount of vitamins and other nutrients, because these techniques use little or no water. In general, the longer and hotter your vegetables cook, and the more water you use, the more nutrients you lose.

Preserving the Nutrient Value of Vegetables and Fruits

▲ Use fresh ingredients whenever possible.
▲ Wash or scrub vegetables and fruits rather than peeling them.
▲ Avoid soaking vegetables or fruits in water.

Vitamin Stability

Some vitamins are more stable than others. Fat-soluble vitamins *stand up to food processing, storage, and cooking better than* water-soluble vitamins. *Vitamin C, for instance, is easily destroyed when exposed to heat, air, oxygen, and light.*

The most unstable vitamins are these:

▲ *Thiamin (vitamin B_1)*

▲ *Vitamin C*

▲ *Folate (folic acid)*

These are more stable vitamins:

▲ *Niacin (vitamin B_3)*

▲ *Biotin (vitamin B_7)*

▲ *Pantothenic acid (vitamin B_5)*

▲ *Vitamin D*

▲ *Vitamin K*

▲ Cut vegetables and fruits into larger pieces; less surface area exposed to air destroys fewer vitamins.

▲ Trim off any roots, separate the leaves (in the case of leafy vegetables), and swish them around in a large bowl of cool water.

▲ Use the outer leaves of vegetables like cabbage or lettuce, unless they are wilted, in which case use them to make vegetable broth.

▲ Remove tough or inedible stems and midribs from vegetables; use them to make vegetable broth.

▲ Dry greens well in paper towels or a salad spinner if serving them in salads; for cooking, leave them damp.

▲ Microwave, steam, roast, or grill vegetables rather than boiling them.

▲ Keep heating times short and cook vegetables until tender-crisp, not soft.

▲ If you boil vegetables, save the nutrient-laden water for soup stock. Use for soups, sauces, stews, or vegetable juices.

▲ Cooking vegetables *quickly* preserves their color as well as their nutrients and helps prevent them from releasing unpleasant odors.

Alternatives to Boiling Vegetables

Steam: Steam vegetables whole or coarsely chopped, either in a vegetable steamer or in a heavy, covered skillet with a quarter to a half inch of water. Make sure the lid is on very tight. However, the lid should be left off cabbage-family vegetables for five to ten minutes before covering them, to allow the sulfur to escape. (Tender greens steam quickly in just the water that clings to the leaves after washing.) If you are planning on sautéing or braising vegetables after steaming, cook them until they are wilted or barely tender. (*Blanching* is the same as boiling, though for a shorter time, and tends to waste more nutrients than steaming or microwaving.) Cooking time: two minutes to thirty minutes.

Microwave: Before sautéing or braising, place washed, but not dried, vegetables in a microwaveable dish; cover loosely and cook until tender. Studies have found that microwaving destroys some antioxidants, according to the *Journal of the Science of Food and Agriculture.*[33] Researchers say that adding a few drops of water before microwaving may help preserve more antioxidants, but this lowers the temperature.[34] Cooking time: four to fifteen minutes.

Sauté: Sauté steamed or microwaved vegetables quickly in a small amount of oil. Season with chopped garlic, onions, leeks, or spices. Cooking time: three to fifteen minutes.

Braising: After sautéing, braising can add tenderness. Add a little broth, cover the pan, and continue cooking the vegetables, then uncover the pan and cook, stirring, until the liquid evaporates. Cooking time: ten to thirty minutes.[35]

More Preparation Tips

▲ Handle fruits and vegetables carefully to avoid bruising, which hastens vitamin C loss.

▲ Cut up produce just before use.

▲ Drain, but do not rinse, pasta after cooking it, because rinsing flushes away nutrients.

▲ Cook rice and other grains in the recommended amount of water or broth so none of the nutrients are wasted.

▲ Phytochemicals are more absorbable from cooked tomatoes than from raw tomatoes.

▲ Liquid from cooked meat and poultry is a rich source of B vitamins; after skimming off the fat, serve it with the meat or use it to make gravy soup.

Food Safety

▲ Wash your hands in hot, soapy water before preparing food. Wash cutting boards, knives, utensils, and countertops in hot, soapy water after preparing each food item and before going on to the next one.

▲ Use one cutting board for raw meat products and another for salads and other foods that are ready to be eaten. To keep flavors unadulterated, it is also a good idea to use one cutting board for savory foods (garlic, vegetables, meat, onions, etc.) and another for fruit and dessert items.

▲ Hot foods should be refrigerated within two hours after cooking. Do not keep the food if it has been standing out for more than two hours. Do not taste-test it, either. Even a small amount of contaminated food can cause illness.

▲ Do not place cooked food on a plate that has held raw meat, poultry, seafood, or uncooked marinades.

▲ Use a meat thermometer to measure the internal temperature of cooked meat and poultry to ensure thorough cooking and avoid bacteria-borne illness. Ground poultry should be cooked to at least 165°F, ground meat to 160°F, roasts and steaks to 145°F, and poultry (whole bird) to 180°F. Boil sauces, soups, and gravy when reheating, and heat other leftovers to 165°F.

CHAPTER NINE

Eating Fit While Eating Out

No question about it—Americans are on the go and eating away from home more than ever before. Many grab a nosh as they zoom between home and work. Professionals eat on the job with business associates, turning meeting times to mealtimes. Time-constrained working parents depend on restaurants to supply what they haven't the energy to provide. Single people often prefer take-out dining to cooking for one. As a consequence, restaurant food is no longer just special-occasion food; it is survival.

Forty-five percent of U.S. food dollars are now spent eating out, according to the National Restaurant Association. The group estimates that within the next ten years, that figure will surpass 53 percent.[36] One in four people eats fast food at least once a day. Unfortunately, most fast food is higher in calories, sodium, and fat and lower in vitamins and minerals than food prepared at home. Even non-fast-food restaurant meals are usually richer, saltier, and more sugary, with portions that challenge you to eat more than you might at home.[37]

Now you know the importance of eating well. But how are you supposed to do this when your schedule is so demanding that you are hardly ever at home?

It is not impossible to achieve a healthy diet, even on the run. In fact, it is easy. Commit to developing the skills to make healthy choices now. It may take time and discipline to turn around bad habits in an environment that promotes so much junk food, but your body will thank you later. You do not have to eat perfectly all the time. As long as your diet is generally good, you can indulge yourself every once in a while.

Make Good Restaurant Choices

Fortunately, America's health consciousness is growing and so, too, is the number of healthful restaurants. Five questions will help you qualify and order restaurant food:

1. How healthy are the *ingredients*?

2. How healthy are the *cooking methods*?

3. How moderate are the *portion sizes*?

4. Do they have *low-fat dishes*?

5. Are food requests *cooked to order*?

Develop a personal list of convenient restaurants that feature the following:

▲ Locally grown produce

▲ Organic lean meat, poultry, fish, and produce

▲ Whole-grain breads and dishes

▲ Fresh, as opposed to processed, food

▲ An "A" rating, signifying outstanding cleanliness

▲ Salads, vegetables, and fruits prepared on-site instead of using previously prepared produce in packages

▲ Grilled, baked, or broiled food, rather than fried

▲ Food cooked using canola or olive oil, not animal fat

▲ Healthy versions of fast-food favorites—pizza and burgers

▲ Low-sodium, low-fat, low-cholesterol dishes, which may be marked with a heart symbol or similar icon

---

Questions to Ask
at Restaurants

1. How do you cook your food? *Fried chicken or fish can soak up three times the fat found in a steak or chop. Broiled, steamed, poached, boiled, baked, or stir-fried dishes are preferable.*

2. What type of fat do you use during preparation? *Saturated fats can increase blood cholesterol levels, so the use of unsaturated oils (see the Oils Group discussion in Chapter 4) is better than using butter, cream, and lard.*

3. Which cuts of meat do you offer? *In addition to seafood and poultry, ask for lean roasts and steaks with visible fat trimmed (see the Meat and Beans Group discussion in Chapter 4.)*

4. Does the dish come with dressing, sauce, or added butter? *If so, ask that it be served on the side. Even salad dressing may contain as many as 200 calories per serving.*

If you cannot tell from the menu whether the restaurant operates this way, do not be shy about asking.

You may want to call a restaurant beforehand to find out whether they will accommodate your requests for healthful food preparation. Even if they will not, customer pressure may eventually force them to change their ways.

Make Good Food Choices

Books like *Fast Food Nation* by Eric Schlosser and Morlon Spurlock's documentary *Super Size Me* are having an effect. Pressure from nutritionists, the media, the government, and consumers themselves is obliging even fast-food restaurants to broaden their menus to include healthier fare. Now you must discipline yourself to forgo the fries and choose the healthier items these restaurants offer. Good food may be more expensive in some cases, but eating less can provide more nutrition if you make sound choices. Ultimately, doing this will save you money because you will eat less, feel better, and avoid costly health consequences. Whether in fast-food or regular restaurants, ask for these:

▲ Salads and vegetables

▲ Sauces and salad dressings on the side (use them sparingly)

▲ Low-cal salad dressings, or oil and vinegar

▲ Clear, rather than cream-based, soups

▲ Salsa and mustard instead of mayonnaise

▲ Olive oil instead of butter

▲ Whole-grain crackers, breads, and side dishes (use side dishes as entrées)

▲ Alternative sources of protein, such as peanut butter, hummus, lentils, or beans

▲ Nonfat or low-fat milk instead of whole milk or cream in your coffee or tea

▲ Fruit juice, nonfat/low-fat milk, or water instead of milk shakes, sodas, or alcoholic beverages

▲ Baked, broiled, or grilled (not fried) *lean* meats including skinless turkey or chicken, beef, and seafood

▲ Fresh fruit or low-fat yogurt instead of rich, sugary desserts

Avoid Unhealthy Choices

High-fat meats, potatoes, side dishes, condiments, and desserts quickly turn a meal into a "heart-stopper." A sugary drink sabotages what is otherwise a healthy offering. Particularly unhealthy choices include these:

▲ Croissant breakfast sandwiches

▲ Danish pastries, coffee cakes, and doughnuts

▲ Fried fish

▲ Fried chicken

▲ Fried eggs

▲ French fries

▲ Onion rings

▲ Fatty-meat (salami, pepperoni, sausage) pizzas

▲ Prepared salads at salad bars such as egg salad, chicken salad, and tuna salad

▲ Fatty cold cuts, such as bologna and salami

▲ Mayonnaise and rich salad dressings

▲ Sodas (large sodas have as many as 300 calories, all empty)

▲ Rich desserts

If you crave foods like these, you should consider them part of your discretionary calories. They are heavier on calories than on nutrients. If you succumb to junk food, try to balance it with healthier foods the rest of that day and the next.

Order Smaller Portions

Calories add up. Excessive portions can cripple your efforts to keep within calorie allotments. Supersizes may make you feel you are getting a lot for your money, but the trade-off is probably poor nutrient value and unnecessary calories. To curb your craving, always refer to the food group recommendations and portions. Keeping the My Pyramid Worksheet with you at all times helps.

Eat Regularly

Eat three times a day, and eat slowly. Many people skip breakfast or lunch in order to "save up" calories for a later large restaurant dinner. Almost invariably this leads to a midmorning or midafternoon slump that can only be satisfied by a Danish, a candy bar, or some other calorie-intensive fix. Even if you tough it out until evening, the famine will leave you ravenous and lead to overordering and overeating food you will then sleep on. Starting the morning with whole grains will supply much-needed nutrients and fuel you through until lunchtime.

Do not munch in the car, on the bus or train, or when walking, standing, or talking on the phone. This "unconscious" eating will keep you from accurate portion counting and good, nutritious meals. Eating slowly helps digestion and makes the most of each mouthful.

▲ Do not supersize your meals.

▲ Order an appetizer, soup, or salad only, instead of an entrée.

▲ Share entrées with a friend or family member.

▲ Eat only half and take the other half home to eat for another meal.

▲ Drink lots of water or other clear, low-cal liquids.

▲ If you must have a dessert, share it with a friend or family member.

▲ At buffets, heap on the whole grains, vegetables, and fruits and take it easy on potato and other starch dishes, meats, sauces, and rich desserts.

Healthful Restaurant Breakfast Foods

▲ *Low-fat whole-grain cereals*

▲ *Low-fat muffins*

▲ *Oatmeal*

▲ *Whole-wheat pancakes or waffles, with fruit yogurt*

▲ *Whole fruit (for fiber)*

▲ *Whole-wheat toast or bagels with ricotta or low-fat cottage cheese and jam*

▲ *Poached or soft-boiled eggs*

▲ *Low-fat yogurt*

Fast, Healthful Lunch Choices

▲ *Single slice of veggie pizza*

▲ *Grilled, not fried, sandwiches*

▲ *Small grilled hamburger on whole-wheat bun*

▲ *Bean burrito*

▲ *Baked potato*

▲ *Side salad with clear dressing*

▲ *Frozen yogurt*

The Ethnic Option

International cuisines usually depend less on protein and more on complex carbohydrates than we do in the United States. This is the very prescription My Pyramid recommends. Consequently, you may have your best luck meeting dietary requirements at ethnic restaurants. Moreover, ethnic foods are sometimes more affordable.

Japanese cuisine is largely fatless, featuring soybean-based foods, lots of rice and noodles, steamed or stir-fried vegetables, and smaller portions of fish and meat. Steer clear of fried tempura, agemono, furai, and katsu dishes. To limit your sodium intake, do not use too much soy sauce, or use low-sodium soy sauce instead.

Chinese specialties are full of vegetables, rice, and noodles, again with smaller meat, poultry, and fish portions. Choose stir-fried or steamed dishes instead of deep-fried items like egg rolls. Since dishes are usually made to order, you can ask that the kitchen use a minimum of oil and no MSG (monosodium glutamate). Again, go light on the soy sauce, or use low-sodium soy sauce.

Thai cooking, like Japanese and Chinese, is rich with vegetables, tofu, rice, and noodles and uses animal protein sparingly. Some of the curry dishes feature coconut milk, which has some saturated fat and should be eaten in moderation.

Indian restaurants offer delicious *dahl*, lentil dishes that substitute for animal protein; flavorful curries; and rice. Tandoor dishes are baked in clay ovens and are usually low-fat. Stay away from fried breads, foods fried in *ghee* (clarified butter), and too much coconut milk.

Mexican food requires some discernment. Forgo the chips and fried foods such as taquitos and chimichangas. Focus on offerings that use peppers, cilantro, and tomatoes instead of sour cream and *con queso* (cheese) fillings. Order black beans instead of refried beans. Go light on the guacamole.

Greek cuisine features the heart-friendly olive oil, but you will have to see your way past the deep-fried appetizers and butter-rich filo dough dishes. Greek baked dishes tend to be full of cream, cheese, and meat, so it is better to order a big Greek salad, grilled fish or lamb, and roasted potatoes.

Italian and *French* food can be an obstacle course for calorie counters, but they are not without healthful resources. Stay away from cream soups and sauces and breaded menu options.

Tip: Take stock of your commitment to health before going into a restaurant. *Visualize the menu and give yourself a pep talk about sticking to healthful foods, cooking methods, and portions. Have a strategy for achieving a balanced but still scrumptious meal.*

Concentrate on food preparations that are baked, grilled, broiled, or steamed. If you have the opportunity, ask that food be sautéed in wine or olive oil instead of butter. Go easy on the bread, which is usually made from refined grains.

Minimize Cocktail-Hour Damage

If there is any way to avoid cocktail hour, do so. Alcoholic drinks have empty calories and can undermine your willpower. In addition, you may find yourself surrounded by a tempting array of high-fat, high-calorie cocktail nibbles and happy-hour food. These are designed to build your thirst, but they do so by sabotaging your diet . . . as well as your cardiovascular well-being. Just to give you an idea, a fist-size helping of fried calamari, even without aioli, is around 500 calories, and a couple dozen nacho chips with cheese can add up to 1,500 calories. Like most cocktail food, these are also loaded with saturated fat.

If cocktail hour is unavoidable, save calories and keep from getting tipsy by choosing lower-calorie, lower-fat mixers such as club soda, sparkling water, or orange, lime, lemon, cranberry, vegetable, or tomato juice. Instead of cocktail food, see if you can get a plate of raw veggies or a shrimp cocktail.

Record Everything You Eat

Keeping comprehensive lists of everything you eat is a hassle, but the discipline will help avert crimes against your calorie allotment. Having the My Pyramid Worksheet on hand will discipline you to eat better food in smaller portions.

CHAPTER TEN

Achieving Peak Nutrition

Tweaking the Pyramid

What if you do everything My Pyramid says and still gain or lose weight? What if you follow the pyramid prescription religiously and you feel sluggish and unwell? Please review the following checklist.

My Pyramid Checklist

▲ Always buy the best, freshest food, organic if possible.

▲ Store and prepare food according to the guidelines in Chapter 8.

▲ Eat enough from each of the six food groups for your activity level.

▲ Eat a broad variety of the best organically cultivated foods.

▲ Do not eat more food than you need to sustain your activity level.

▲ Do not eat excess saturated fat, sodium, or added sugar.

▲ Exercise for at least thirty minutes daily.

▲ Get plenty of sleep.

▲ Minimize exposure to stress and pollution.

Has complying with all of these recommendations not stabilized your weight and improved your well-being? Then carefully monitor your activity level to determine whether you need to adjust your calorie intake. Whereas naturally nervous people generally metabolize food faster, more relaxed types simply do not burn calories as easily. If you are losing weight on the My Pyramid regime and don't need to, try eating more. If you are gaining weight and don't need to, try eating fewer calories. Either way, do not sacrifice nutrients no matter what. Do not skimp on the requirements for whole grains, vegetables, and fruit.

Nutritional Supplements

The best way for us to get our nutrients is by eating plenty of *whole foods.* Whole foods—such as unprocessed fruits, vegetables, and whole grains—provide a complex combination of vitamins, minerals, fiber, and other substances that promote health. This complex chemistry delivers the essential vitamins, minerals, and trace elements, and ensures that they are absorbed. No supplement can take the place of nutritious food—and that is one reason My Pyramid does not cover the subject—but as this book makes clear, eating a healthy, well-balanced diet is increasingly difficult. Many people either cannot or do not eat enough high-quality food. Pregnant women and older adults have unique nutritional needs that are even more difficult to meet.

Therefore, if you have trouble getting enough nutrients, you may benefit from taking a high-quality, complete multi-vitamin-mineral supplement. Though supplements cannot replicate all of the nutrients and benefits of whole foods, they can complement your diet and make up for deficient foods. Taking a supplement can easily become habit-forming in the best sense. Supplements are added insurance.

To use supplements safely, first . . .

▲ Weigh your nutritional needs

▲ Assess the merits of taking a supplement

▲ Understand how to choose and use dietary supplements

When choosing a nutritional supplement *do not substitute quality for cost*. Purchase supplements in a form that is absorbable; otherwise, the supplement is a waste of money.

Read the label carefully, including the fine print. Product labels state the active ingredients, which nutrients are included, the serving size, and the amount of nutrients in each serving. The label also provides directions for safe use and tips for storage. You will find the name and address

How Much Should You Get Each Day?

No two people's nutrient needs are the same. Following are minimum adult requirements.

Nutrient	Amount
Biotin	300 mcg
Calcium	1,000 mg
Chloride	3,400 mg
Chromium	120 mcg
Copper	2 mg
Folic acid	400 mcg
Iodine	150 mcg
Iron	18 mg
Magnesium	400 mg
Manganese	2 mg
Molybdenum	75 mcg
Niacin	20 mg
Pantothenic acid	10 mg
Phosphorus	1,000 mg
Riboflavin	1.7 mg
Selenium	70 mcg
Thiamin	1.5 mg
Vitamin A	5,000 IU
Vitamin B$_6$	2 mg
Vitamin B$_{12}$	6 mcg
Vitamin C	60 mg
Vitamin D	400 IU

(continued)

Vitamin E	30 IU
Vitamin K	80 mcg
Zinc	15 mg
Total fat	65 g
Saturated fat	20 g
Cholesterol	300 mg
Total carbohydrate	300 g
Fiber	25 g
Sodium	2,400 mg
Potassium	3,500 mg
Protein	50 g

Source: Center for Food Safety and Applied Nutrition, 2002; National Academy of Sciences.

of the manufacturer, packer, or distributor to whom you can write if you need more information.

Choose a multi-vitamin-mineral supplement that provides about 100 Percent Daily Value (% DV; see Chapter 7) of all the vitamins and minerals, instead of one that supplies megadoses of one vitamin and only 20% DV of another. Nutrient toxicity can result from high-dose supplements. Less expensive supplements sometimes do not contain the more expensive nutrients—such as vitamin E—in a quantity sufficient to meet the 100% DV. The exception to this is calcium, because 100% DV of calcium would make a tablet too large to swallow.

Make sure "USP" appears on the label. The testing organization U.S. Pharmacopeia certifies that nutritional supplements meet strength, purity, disintegration, and dissolution health standards.

Check the expiration date, since supplements lose potency over time. If a supplement does not have an expiration date, do not buy it. Discard those that have expired.

Store all vitamin and mineral supplements safely in a dry, cool place, away from children. Iron overdose is a leading cause of poisoning deaths among children. Avoid hot, humid storage locations, such as the bathroom.

Take supplements with meals, to maximize absorption.

Special health concerns may generate a need for additional or different vitamins or minerals. There is some controversy over whether all nutrients should be supplied at the

100% DV level. For example, a risk of osteoporosis can double the vitamin A requirement, but too much vitamin A can be toxic. Vitamin K is more important to those who have been on antibiotics.[38] Supplemental vitamin E can be dangerous for individuals on anticoagulants.[39] *Specific health issues make it essential to consult a qualified physician, pharmacist, and/or registered dietitian concerning the use of any dietary supplements.*

Seeking Professional Nutritional Care

If following My Pyramid's advice, including taking a supplement, and adjusting your intake do not improve your health, you must look for additional help. It may be either that you are ill or that you been exposed to more stress or poorer environmental conditions than your body can accommodate. Typical nutrition-related problems that can be alleviated with better nutrition but may require help from a nutritional professional are as follows:

▲ Weight gain or loss

▲ Food allergies

▲ Fatigue and chronic fatigue syndrome

▲ Digestive disorders

▲ Gastrointestinal trouble, including irritable bowel syndrome

▲ Headaches, migraines

▲ *Candida albicans*

▲ Nutritional imbalances

▲ Food cravings

▲ Arthritis

▲ High blood pressure

▲ Cardiovascular problems

▲ Blood sugar imbalances and diabetes

▲ Anorexia and bulimia

Obviously, some of these are potentially severe conditions that require a physician's care in addition to a nutritionist's program.

A nutrition professional may be able to help you. Registered dietitians must have a bachelor's degree in nutrition—which includes the study of physiology, anatomy, biochemistry, biology, chemistry, and nutrition—and nine hundred hours of supervised practice. They must have passed a national registration exam. Even more knowledgeable are registered dietitians at a master's degree or PhD level. The most experienced are fellows of the American Dietetic Association; they have the initials "FADA" after their name.

To find a nutritionist, ask your physician for a recommendation or check the Yellow Pages of the phone book. You may also find the names and numbers of qualified nutrition professionals throughout the United States by calling the American Dietetic Association's Nutrition Information Line, 1-800-366-1655. This information can be found on the Internet at www.eatright.org.

Before your visit, ask the nutritionist specific questions:

1. What is your philosophy regarding diet and nutrition?

2. Do you have a nutritional specialty?

3. Where did you train?

4. What are your degrees and professional credentials?

5. What is your process for making a diagnosis?

6. What kinds of treatment plans do you recommend?

7. How often will I need to consult with you?

8. How much does a session cost?

9. Are your services covered by medical insurance?

10. Will you or someone else conduct the treatment? If someone else, will you supervise the treatment?

11. What are the alternative treatments?

12. What are the benefits and the risks associated with the recommended treatment? With the alternative treatments?

13. What role do family members or friends play in a particular treatment?

This conversation should confirm the practitioner's professionalism and give you a sense of whether you can communicate openly with him or her. Issues related to diet are usually very personal, and the ability to express yourself without reservation is extremely important.

What to Expect

After assessing your nutrition status related to your health condition, nutritionists devise a plan for incorporating the right kinds of foods and supplemental nutrients to address your health issues. A nutritionist will also recommend exercise as a companion to a dietary regimen as appropriate.

Typically, nutritionists recommend the best quality of food available; the regimen will probably have much in common with My Pyramid. You may be asked to keep a food diary, but if you have been using the My Pyramid worksheet, you will be used to this.

The lessons of My Pyramid persist. The wrong foods can make you ill, but good food really can improve your health. Whether or not it takes professional help to tailor a diet to your medical issues, committing to My Pyramid can revolutionize your outlook and your life.

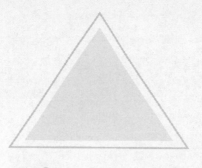

Afterword

Developments in food and eating never end. Nutritional research will continue to supply more information in more detail. In fact, researchers are at work right now in a brand-new field called *nutrigenomics,* which may eventually lead to an even more personalized food pyramid. Industry will turn out a bigger selection of newfangled foodstuffs. And nutritionists and physicians will unveil yet more new diets. At the same time, environmental degradation will probably increase even as our population multiplies, which may compromise and limit food supplies.

You, the consumer, are not helpless. By educating yourself, being a savvy shopper, and insisting on the freshest, healthiest groceries, you help ensure that good sense and technology will respond, fostering our access to delicious, nutrient-rich foods. Demand the best. You deserve it. Good luck and *bon appetit!*

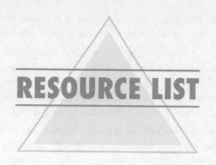

RESOURCE LIST

Organizations and Websites

The official My Pyramid website: **www.mypyramid.gov. U.S. Department of Agriculture:** www.usda.gov, 1400 Independence Ave. S.W., Washington, DC 20250.

Center for Nutrition Policy and Promotion: www.cnpp.usda.gov, c/o U.S. Department of Agriculture, 1400 Independence Ave. S.W., Washington, DC 20250, 703-305-7600.

Slow Food U.S.A. is an educational organization dedicated to stewardship of the land and ecologically sound food production. www.slowfoodusa.org, 20 Jay Street, Suite 313, Brooklyn, NY 11201, 718-260-8000.

Nutrispeak.com specializes in vegetarian nutrition and food sensitivities.

Eatwild.com tells where and why to get safe, healthy, natural, and nutritious grass-fed beef, lamb, goats, bison, poultry, and dairy products.

Sustainable Table helps direct consumers to the leading organizations that are working on sustainable food issues. www.sustainabletable.org/home/, c/o Global Resource Action Center for the Environment (GRACE), 215 Lexington Ave, Suite 1001, New York, NY 10016, 212-726-9161.

Stay informed about all sides of the latest medical news and health information and discover how to prevent disease, optimize health and weight, and live longer by subscribing to a free newsletter at **www.mercola.com.** Mercola Fulfillment Center, 1600 South 4650 West, Salt Lake City, UT 84104.

Local Harvest lists the freshest, healthiest, most flavorful organic food grown closest to you. Use the website to find farmers markets, family farms, and other sources of sustainably grown food in your area, where you can buy produce, grass-fed meats, and many other goodies. www.localharvest.org, 220 21st Ave., Santa Cruz, CA 95062, 831-475-8150.

The Organic Center for Education and Promotion provides consumers, health care professionals, educators, public officials, and government agencies with credible, scientific information about the organic benefit. www.organic-center.org, 46 East Killingly Road, Foster, RI 02825, 401-647-1502.

Community Food Security Coalition is dedicated to building strong, sustainable local and regional food systems that ensure access to affordable, nutritious, and culturally appropriate food for all people at all times. Its excellent website has links to many nutrition organizations and farmers market groups. www.foodsecurity.org/links.html#nutrition, P.O. Box 209, Venice, CA 90294, 310-822-5410.

Food and Nutrition Information Center, www.nutrition.gov, 10301 Baltimore Avenue, Beltsville, MD 20705-2351, 301-504-5755.

Food Technology and Safety, 10301 Baltimore Avenue, Beltsville, MD 20705-2351, 301-504-8400.

American Dietetic Association, www.eatright.org, 120 South Riverside Plaza, Suite 2000, Chicago, IL 60606-6995, 800-877-1600, Nutrition Information Line, 1-800-366-1655.

Center for Food Safety and Applied Nutrition, Food and Drug Administration, www.cfsan.fda.gov/list.html, 5100 Paint Branch Parkway, College Park, MD 20740-3835, 888-SAFEFOOD.

How to Read the Label of a Nutritional Supplement, www.pioneernutritional.com/pdfs/readlabelposter.pdf.

Books

Carole C. Baldwin and Julie H. Mounts, *One Fish, Two Fish, Crawfish, Bluefish: The Smithsonian Sustainable Seafood Cookbook* (Smithsonian Books, 2003).

Kelly D. Brownell, PhD, *Food Fight: The Inside Story of the Food Industry, America's Obesity Crisis and What We Can Do About It* (McGraw-Hill, 2003).

Greg Critser, *Fat Land: How Americans Became the Fattest People in the World* (Houghton Mifflin, 2003).

Lavon J. Dunne, *Nutrition Almanac* (McGraw-Hill, 2001).

Elson M. Haas, M.D., *Staying Healthy with Nutrition: The Complete Guide to Diet and Nutritional Medicine* (Celestial Arts, 1992).

Brian Halweil, *Eat Here: Homegrown Pleasures in a Global Supermarket* (Norton, 2004).

Frances Moore Lappé, *Diet for a Small Planet* (Ballantine, 1985).

Deborah Madison and Edward Espe Brown, *The Greens Cookbook* (Broadway, 2001).

Deborah Madison, *Local Flavors: Cooking and Eating from America's Farmers' Markets* (Broadway, 2002).

Deborah Madison, *This Can't Be Tofu!: 75 Recipes to Cook Something You Never Thought You Would—and Love Every Bite* (Broadway, 2000).

Susan Mitchell, PhD, RD, FADA, and Catherine Christie, PhD, RD, FADA, *Fat Is Not Your Fate: Outsmart Your Genes and Lose Weight Forever* (Fireside, 2004).

Marion Nestle, *Food Politics: How the Food Industry Influences Nutrition and Health* (California Studies in Food and Culture, 3) (University of California Press, 2003).

Leon Rappoport, *How We Eat: Appetite, Culture, and the Psychology of Food* (ECW Press, 2003).

Eric Schlosser, *Fast Food Nation: The Dark Side of the All-American Meal* (Houghton Mifflin, 2001).

Joanne Stepaniak and Vesanto Melina, *Raising Vegetarian Children: A Guide to Good Health and Family Harmony* (McGraw-Hill, 2002).

Norman Wirzba, *The Essential Agrarian Reader: The Future of Culture, Community, and the Land* (Shoemaker & Hoard, 2004).

Magazines

Alternative Medicine

Cooking Light

Eating Well

Living Without

Prevention and Prevention.com

Saveur

Slow

The Snail

Vegetarian Times

Newsletters

Berkeley Wellness Letter

Consumer Reports on Health

Environmental Nutrition

Tufts University Health & Nutrition Letter

Publications

Dietary Guidelines for Americans, 2005, available online at www.mypyramid
.gov, or directly through the USDA (address listed under "Organizations
and Websites").

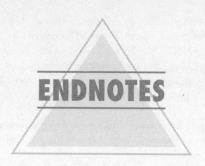

ENDNOTES

1. Annual Deaths Attributable to Obesity in the United States, http://jama.ama-assn.org/cgi/content/abstract/282/16/1530.
2. Comparative Causes of Annual Deaths, Centers for Disease Control, http://www.cdc.gov/tobacco/research_data/health_consequences/andths.htm.
3. National Diabetes Fact Sheet, American Diabetes Association, http://www.diabetes.org/diabetes-statistics/national-diabetes-fact-sheet.jsp.
4. National Institute of Diabetes and Digestive and Kidney Diseases, http://diabetes.niddk.nih.gov/dm/pubs/statistics/#7.
5. National Center for Health Statistics, http://www.cdc.gov/nchs/fastats/hyprtens.htm.
6. Prevalence and Incidence of Heart Disease, http://www.wrongdiagnosis.com/c/cholesterol/prevalence.htm.
7. Your Digestive System and How It Works, http://digestive.niddk.nih.gov/ddiseases/pubs/yrdd/.
8. Dietary Reference Intakes, http://www.iom.edu/Object.File/Master/7/300/0.pdf.
9. http://atoz.iqhealth.com/HealthAnswers/encyclopedia/HTMLfiles/2935.html.
10. http://www.mindfully.org/Food/Irradiation-USDA-Approved22oct02.htm.

11. http://www.betterhealthchannel.com.au/bhcv2/bhcarticles.nsf/pages/ Food_processing_and_nutrition?OpenDocument.

12. Junk Food: How Much Can You Get Away With?, http:// www.pdrhealth.com/content/nutrition_health/chapters/fgnt37.shtml.

13. Daryn Eller, "Original Food" *Natural Health,* October 2003, http://www .findarticles.com/p/articles/mi_m0NAH/is_8_33/ai_108786006#continue.

14. *National Report on Human Exposure to Environmental Chemicals,* Centers for Disease Control, http://www.cdc.gov/exposurereport/2nd/ introduction.htm.

15. http://www.cdc.gov/nccdphp/sgr/ataglan.htm.

16. Amanda Gardner, Mental Disorders on the Rise in the United States, http://www.depressionissues.com/ms/news/521923/main.html.

17. Brendan I. Koerner, Disorders Made to Order July/August 2002, http://www.motherjones.com/news/feature/2002/07/disorders.html.

18. *Dietary Guidelines for Americans, 2005,* Chapter 5, http://www.health .gov/dietaryguidelines/dga2005/document/html/chapter5.htm.

19. Elson M. Haas, M.D., *Staying Healthy with Nutrition,* Celestial Arts, 1992, page 315.

20. Understanding Free Radicals and Antioxidants, http://www .healthchecksystems.com/antioxid.htm.

21. Ibid.

22. http://us.cambridge.org/Books/kiple/lactose.htm.

23. The Properties of Milk, http://www.wholisticresearch.com/info/ artshow.php3?artid=22.

24. USDA, *Dietary Guidelines for Americans, 2005.*

25. United Nations University Press, *Food and Nutrition Bulletin,* volume 17, number 3, September 1996. Amino acid composition of food groups, http://www.unu.edu/unupress/food/8F173e/8F173E09.htm#Amino- %20acid%20composition%20of%20food%20groups, Massachusetts Nutrient Data Bank

26. Nutrition Research, Inc., *The Nutrition Almanac,* McGraw-Hill, 1984.

27. Elizabeth Vierck and Kris Hodges, *Aging: Demographics, Health, and Health Services,* Greenwood Press, 2003.

28. The Renaissance of Fat: Roles in Membrane Structure, Signal Transduction and Gene Expression, http://www.mja.com.au/public/issues/ 176_11_030602/S109-S110.html.

29. http://www.fda.gov/fdac/features/2003/503_fats.html.

30. Rutgers University and Community Food Security Coalition, North American Initiative on Urban Agriculture.

31. Carol B. Suter, *Nutrient Retention in Vegetables.*

32. http://www.lesliebeck.com/transcript.php?tid=296.

33. myhealth.chh.org/healthyliving/nutrition/jul04nutritionmicrowave.htm.

34. http://www.lesliebeck.com/transcript.php?tid=296.

35. http://nutrition.lifetips.com/cat/23565/preserving-nutrients/.

36. The Secrets to Healthy Restaurant Eating, http://www.pdrhealth.com/content/nutrition_health/chapters/fgnt38.shtml.

37. Fast Food Nutrition, http://www.helpguide.org/aging/fast_food_nutrition.htm.

38. Choosing a Multi-Vitamin Mineral Supplement, James M. Gerber, http://www.nnfa-northwest.com/documents/health/vitamin.htm.

39. Mayo Clinic Staff, Vitamin and Mineral Supplements, Use with Care, http://www.mayoclinic.com/invoke.cfm?id=NU00198.

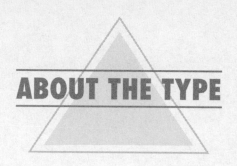

ABOUT THE TYPE

This book was set in Galliard, a typeface designed by Matthew Carter for the Mergenthaler Linotype Company in 1978. Galliard is based on the sixteenth-century typefaces of Robert Granjon.